THE MO............K
A WOMAN CAN READ

This groundbreaking book covers every aspect of a woman's sexual development. Here is the most up-to-date information about:

- puberty
- menstruation
- menstrual irregularities
- contraception
- conception
- toxic shock syndrome
- premenstrual syndrome (PMS)
- menopause

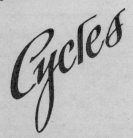

A MENSTRUAL GUIDE FOR WOMEN OF ALL AGES

The book that answers the questions asked by women who want to understand their bodies.

Cycles:

EVERY WOMAN'S GUIDE TO MENSTRUATION

by Patricia Allen, M.D. and Denise Fortino

PINNACLE BOOKS

NEW YORK

CYCLES: EVERY WOMAN'S GUIDE TO MENSTRUATION

Copyright © 1983 by Patricia Allen, M.D. and Denise Fortino

An original Pinnacle Books edition, published for the first time anywhere.

First printing, December 1983

ISBN: 0-523-42145-1

Printed in the United States of America

PINNACLE BOOKS, INC.
1430 Broadway
New York, New York 10018

9 8 7 6 5 4 3 2 1

This book is dedicated to our mothers, whom we love and admire deeply.

The authors wish to thank Nina Finkelstein, former editor at *Ms.*, for her careful reading and thoughtful comments.

CONTENTS

CYCLES:
EVERY WOMAN'S GUIDE TO MENSTRUATION

Chapter 1

TRACING THE MENSTRUAL CYCLE

Every month, from about your early teens to late middle age, your body is under the sway of *cycles*—urged on by its own powerful hormones to enact the ritual of reproduction. Secreted in a rise-and-fall sequence by pea-sized glands, mere droplets of these chemical messengers are duty-bound by orders issued from your brain to regulate the organs of fertility and respond to their signals in turn. Whether or not you have a baby, your body, poised with potential energy, will go through the motions anyway, tirelessly rehearsing and readying itself for the main event.

"Periods" are simply visible proof of this monthly, all-out effort. They are also, as one doctor observes, a reminder that the tempo of cyclical change, carefully clocked and controlled, is what makes the female body tick for much of a lifetime: A monthly chart of our primary hormones, estrogen and progesterone, would look like the Dow Jones Industrial Average.[1]

In their endless ebb and flow, women's cycles may sometimes mimic one another, persuading bodies to operate in sync: Thus, studies have shown that the menstrual rhythms of those who share living space for an extended time may ultimately occur simultaneously. And our cycles exert other influences as well—upon emotions, mood, even sex drive. Not long ago, a report published in *The New England Journal of Medicine* suggested that women are readily aroused and initiate lovemaking more often when they are most fertile and hormone levels are at their highest—during the second phase of the menstrual cycle. Another finding reveals that some men may experience subtle cyclical variations, too: For example, the testosterone (male hormone) levels of married men have been found to increase along with the testosterone present in their wives (which fuels sexual desire), thus challenging the notion that men are biologically changeless.

Your monthly cycle may be reflected in a wider sphere as well. Consider the origin of the word *menstruation*—from the Latin word *mens* meaning month, a derivation of moon. (The Greek word for moon is *mene*.) It did not escape the ancients' notice that the average length of the female cycle is almost identical to the period between two full moons. Some observers still argue that it is difficult to regard the similarity between lunar and menstrual cycles as entirely coincidental. Darwin, pointing to the pattern, speculated that menstruation was related to the action of the moon on tides—a phenomenon connected with man's origins in the sea.[2]

The image of the cycle suggests something timeless and predictable, full of reassuring rhyme and reason. And that's exactly how all women should regard menstruation—as a normal, routine event with its own internal rules of order; nothing arbitrary, mysterious or terribly complicated.

Every healthy woman menstruates: Monthly bleeding is truly one of the body's vital signs—that you are functioning normally and in good condition. In fact, it can be a very revealing barometer of health, as telling an index as your blood pressure or resting heart rate. The monthly cycle itself can generate an astonishing number of changes in your body and mind, including body temperature, heart rhythm, metabolism, the level of nutrients circulating in your blood, changes in breast tissue, even the color and permeability of your skin.

Menstruation signals neither disadvantage nor disability:

2

It is simply silly to describe it in coy, sugar-coated language or disparaging terms. Nor is it unmentionable, to be hidden from friends or family, male or female. And, contrary to lingering myths, sports, exercise and sexual activity are all beneficial any day of the month—menstruation need not bring these to a standstill.

If a woman feels that periods are a sign of illness or a mystery, dirty, demeaning or debilitating, such a view can "adversely affect her body image, her sexuality, dietary habits, even her attitudes toward medication, contraception and family planning," writes Letty Cottin Pogrebin, an editor at *Ms.* and author of *Growing Up Free: Raising Your Child in the 80s* (McGraw-Hill). And while the physical discomforts (experienced by more than half of all menstruating women, according to most estimates) are very *real* complaints with physical origins, studies have found that the power of suggestion may intensify existing distress: What women report about their symptoms may be shaped in part by what they have been led to expect. For example, women who are told they are premenstrual have been found to describe a greater degree of pain, bloating and eating changes than those who are made to believe they are between periods (when in fact the two groups are at the very same phase in their cycles).

The more you know about the female cycle, the better acquainted you will be with your body and how it works. Such knowledge, like any other kind, is power—in this case, the power to safeguard your health in the best possible way. By being a well-informed patient, you can become a responsible participant in any care your doctor provides.

The patients who fill my office every day are inquisitive, thoughtful, self-motivated women who enjoy exchanging ideas, discussing various choices of treatment and learning about their bodies. These women don't seek to dictate medical practice, only to understand it and raise well-reasoned questions of their own. I find them gratifying to

3

work with because they are interested in the quality of life all around—not just their bodies, but their emotional and professional lives as well. Together, our goal is to prevent illness, and when treatment is unavoidable, to achieve the most acceptable results with the fewest possible side effects.

As patients have become more enlightened and educated, so have doctors. If I am more considerate of my patients' needs and feelings, freer of rigid, paternalistic views about women's health care than some gynecologists may have been in the past, it is because times have changed for the better, medical training has become more progressive and humanistic—and I am simply a product of such training.

For most of the women I see, menstruation is not a major problem or a source of unremitting misery. (The vast majority of women are *not* disabled by their periods.) However, the discomforts experienced by many of us, ranging from mild twinges to severe spasmodic pain, are very specific, identifiable, physiological complaints, and not simply the figments of an agitated psyche, as physicians so long assumed. I will discuss dysmenorrhea (painful periods) and its various forms and causes in Chapter II.

MENSTRUATION WITHOUT MYSTERY

To ask intelligent questions or participate in decisions concerning your health, you need to be armed with facts—namely, the ABC's of the menstrual cycle. Awareness of how the cycle works—the ability to visualize the process from start to finish—can tell you so much else about your body: how conception occurs and how to prevent it; the whys of premenstrual syndrome and menstrual cramps; greater insight about menopause, and more. For this reason, it's probably among the most crucial pieces of medical information you ever need to know. Surprisingly, a good many women, perhaps most, would be hard-pressed to describe the full menstrual story in accurate detail without consulting an encyclopedia first.

4

Despite our technical ignorance, for virtually all of us, the very first period stands out in vivid memory. You may recall the exact date and year, even time of day, you began to menstruate. Ask your friends, your mother, and each, too, will promptly tell you just when and where the momentous rite of passage occurred, what she was doing or wearing, how she responded. Chances are the reactions will run the gamut—awe, surprise, embarrassment, delight, disgust, excitement, dread—depending on what she knew or felt about her body at the time, what her own mother had told her. (It's no surprise that a parent's attitude toward menstruation can be profoundly influential.)

Biologically speaking, you might think of this well-remembered first period as actually the *last* of a series of bodily changes—starting at around age seven or eight and collectively known as puberty. Menstruation is the grand climax in this chain of events which generally begins with the budding and enlargement of breasts, followed by the growth of pubic hair, a spurt in height and weight, and a widening of the hips and pelvic bones. In fact, about 90 percent of a young woman's growth has already taken place by the time she begins to menstruate. The average age at the first period or menarche (pronounced menARKY) is now 12.3 in the U.S., and the normal range is anywhere from nine to 16.

But the menstrual cycle can be traced to an even earlier moment, months before you are born. A critical point in an embryo's development determines whether a cluster of specialized nerve cells within its brain (the budding, all-important hypothalamus) will secrete hormones for the rest of its life in a cyclical or constant pattern, that of female or male.[3] The presence of testosterone in the fetal bloodstream means that two crucial hormones, FSH and LH, will issue forth from the hypothalamus in an undeviating rhythm throughout a lifetime. The male body forms not only FSH and LH but also sperm and testosterone at a steady rate. The *absence* of testosterone in a developing embryo will pave the way for the characteristic *cycles* of a woman's reproductive life. Instead of emerging in a constant stream, her hormones will fluctuate; shifting levels of these substances will be playing off against each other at different times of the month, establishing the potential to implant and nourish new life—a pattern that will prevail from menarche to menopause.[4]

HORMONES AND YOUR PERIOD

The hormones that eventually trigger the menstrual cycle actually make their quiet debut about five years *before* menarche. First, a substance called follicle-stimulating hormone (FSH), released by the pituitary gland at the base of the brain, works its subtle influence on certain cells of a young girl's ovaries. Awakened by FSH, these begin churning out the very first traces of the potent hormone estrogen into the bloodstream. Incredibly minute amounts are enough to spur the growth and development of the entire reproductive network over the next few years: stimulating breast tissue, the sprouting of pubic hairs, the enlargement and heightening erotic sensitivity of the vagina, cervix and uterus; the layering of fat on hips, thighs, buttocks and abdomen. Estrogen sculpts the female body inside and out, shaping the contours and curves that ultimately distinguish it from a man's.

By the time a girl is about 11 years old, the amount of FSH in her body has multiplied about sevenfold—and with it, the level of estrogen. Other hormones, from the thyroid, adrenals and pituitary, act in concert with estrogen to enlarge the sexual organs. When she is around 12, the hypothalamus, the region right above the pituitary, starts conducting the hormonal symphony. While carefully monitoring her estrogen level all along, it suddenly detects a significant drop in the hormone as it is consumed by its wide-ranging functions.

In response, the hypothalamus prods the pituitary to secrete more FSH. This now prompts about 20 immature follicles—clusters of cells enveloping the eggs within each ovary—to produce additional estrogen. This time, the hormone stimulates the lining of the uterus, causing it to thicken and start "rehearsing" for the arrival of an egg. The potential for fertility has begun.

A seven-month-old female embryo contains the maximum number of eggs—about half a million—it will ever have. But these microscopic seeds of life start deteriorating soon after: By birth, the ovaries contain only half this amount, and by menarche, the number of eggs has dwindled to about 75,000. Of these, only about 400 to 500 will ripen and find their way to the uterus for possible fertilization, a process called ovulation. Once the menstrual cycle has settled into an orderly rhythm, ovulation occurs in most women about 11 to 13 times a year. That means the typical reproductive or fertile life span numbers between 30 to 40 years.

In any established monthly cycle, the scenario unfolds as follows: During the first two weeks, under the dominant influence of FSH and estrogen, one apparently "chosen" follicle gains supremacy, continuing to ripen and mature as the others wither away. About 14 days later, the hypothalamus, now registering an abundance of estrogen, instructs the pituitary to curb its output of FSH and release increasing amounts of an agent called LH (luteinizing hormone). LH causes the fully ripened egg to burst out of its follicle walls and begin its journey toward the uterus. The scar tissue left in its wake becomes transformed into a temporary gland called the corpus luteum (literally, "yellow body") which manufactures the hormone progesterone. Along with the remaining estrogen, progesterone further enriches and engorges the uterine lining, and, should pregnancy occur, can sustain a growing embryo for the first few months.

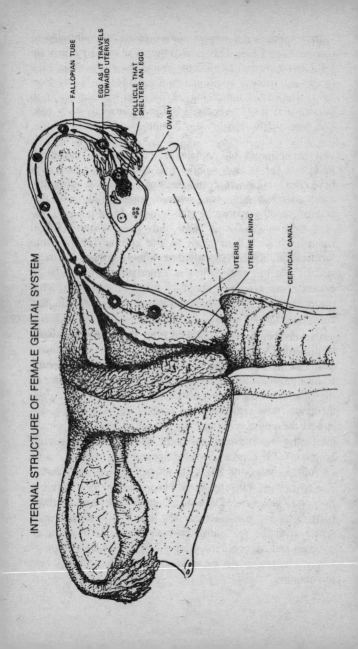

INTERNAL STRUCTURE OF FEMALE GENITAL SYSTEM

FALLOPIAN TUBE

EGG AS IT TRAVELS TOWARD UTERUS

FOLLICLE THAT SHELTERS AN EGG

OVARY

UTERUS

UTERINE LINING

CERVICAL CANAL

If an egg is not fertilized, the hypothalamus will simply order the pituitary to stop releasing FSH and LH, and so reduce the body's output of both estrogen and progesterone—the uterine buildup becomes futile at this point. Without the hormonal stimulus, the corpus luteum shrivels and disappears, and the spongy endometrial tissue begins breaking apart. The resulting mucous, blood and cast-off cells, including the unfertilized egg, flows down via the uterus and cervix, and out through the vagina as menstrual fluid. (In a woman who has not had sexual intercourse, the thin membrane or hymen covering the vaginal opening is normally perforated to permit release of the menstrual matter. Very rarely, a thick and fibrous hymen may block the passage and delay menstruation; minor surgery can correct the problem.)

Just before the menstrual flow appears, as the lining begins breaking down, hormone levels are at their *lowest*. This deficiency alerts the hypothalamus to activate the pituitary, and the entire process occurs anew. Each cycle "officially" starts with the first day of bleeding, so estrogen levels begin rising slowly from this point on, with progesterone joining in at mid-cycle.

To calculate the length of your cycle: Count the interval starting from the first day of one period up to, but not including, the first day of your next. Thus, if your period begins on Sept. 1 and your next one on Sept. 29, your cycle length is 28 days, not 29.

The blood released during menstruation typically amounts to no more than several teaspoons, though its color and (usually non-clotting) consistency may sometimes make it seem like more. While many women report the heaviest discharge on the first two days and a much lighter flow thereafter, others experience the opposite pattern, from scanty to heavy, or sustain the same volume throughout their period—consistently light, moderate *or* substantial.

In the same woman, periods occasionally vary in both length and the amount of blood lost. Those who take birth

9

control pills, for example, may have very light periods, sometimes almost none at all. It is not unusual for IUD wearers to have a much longer and heavier flow, especially during the first few months following insertion. Later on, the bleeding should taper off to a more normal level, though it may still be heavier than it was before insertion of the IUD.

During the first six to 12 cycles of a woman's life, ovulation generally does not occur. (These are called anovulatory periods.) As one physician notes, "It's as if nature puts the young uterus through a few dummy runs before allowing eggs to be launched on their search for a future." Thus, a 12-year-old body is not yet fully equipped to bear and sustain a child—so anovulatory periods may be automatic insurance against premature pregnancy. However, this is by no means an absolute, dependable rule, as many a young mother-to-be can testify!

Failure to ovulate explains why the earliest menstrual cycles are often irregular and relatively free of spasmodic pain. Think of ovulation as the built-in timer of the menstrual process—in about 90 percent of women, the flow occurs between 13 and 15 days after this event. Without egg release, there is no such pacing and periods are more likely to be erratic. As for pain, with only estrogen at work to build up the endometrium, the walls of the uterus aren't as thick as they would be in a normal cycle. This means that substances called *prostaglandins*, which are secreted by the lining of the womb and are responsible for painful muscle contractions, are not produced in their usual abundance.

While a girl's periods may be unpredictable the first year, by the third year of her cycle they generally settle down to a recognizable pattern. The so-called standard cycle is 28 days, though anywhere from 21 to 35 is considered average and the reported normal range is as wide as 21 to 44 days. The length of a cycle is not as important as its consistency. Any abrupt deviation from a

THE AVERAGE 28 DAY MENSTRUAL CYCLE

DEVELOPMENT AND RELEASE OF EGG; BUILDUP OF UTERINE LINING FROM DAY 1-28

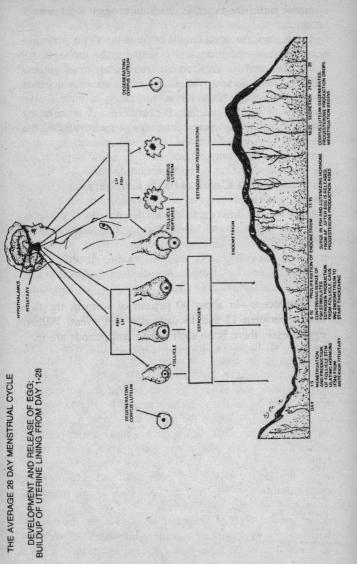

regularly established routine should be brought to a doctor's attention.

To sum up, the adult female cycle refers to the periodic, hormone-regulated process that prepares the uterus to receive and nurture a fertilized egg—a monthly ritual orchestrated by the brain and ovaries. The whole outcome depends on the release and perfect synchronization of microscopic amounts of highly specialized chemicals. If fertilization does not occur, the cycle culminates in menstruation, the shedding of thickened, blood-rich uterine tissue.

THE CYCLE AND ITS CHANGES

Like any other biological clock, the menstrual cycle is delicately balanced and susceptible to many influences: It can be disturbed, delayed or accelerated by emotional stress, physical illness or trauma, nervous disorders, climate and time zone changes, diet, thyroid dysfunction and a host of other factors. (See Chapter III on menstrual irregularities.)

The ups and downs of the cycle correspond to various changes within the body throughout the month, aside from those occurring inside the uterus. One of the most telling variations is the change in the texture of cervical fluid or mucus. During the first half of the cycle, it is very syrupy, thick and elastic, as if to protect the cervix and uterus from bacteria and form a natural barrier to sperm. At ovulation, LH causes the mucus to become thinner and more transparent. This allows sperm a much easier passage so fertilization can take place readily after an egg exits from the ovary. When the egg has completed its journey along the length of the Fallopian tube and progesterone output dominates, the fluid thickens once again, resulting in a kind of built-in "diaphragm." If pregnancy does occur and the level of progesterone stays high, the mucus will become even stickier and more impenetrable, serving to shield the fragile fetus from bacterial invasion.

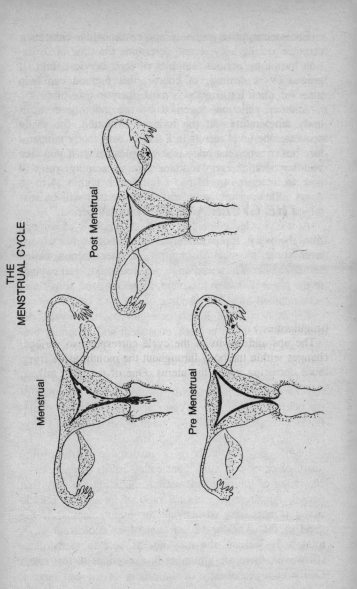

THE MENSTRUAL CYCLE

Menstrual

Pre Menstrual

Post Menstrual

13

For contraceptive purposes, some women can chart their progress during a cycle and determine the time of ovulation by taking periodic samples of their cervical fluid. If pregnancy is desired, of course, this method can help pinpoint when fertilization is most likely to take place.

Another variation governed by the monthly cycle is body temperature. At the time of ovulation, the rising progesterone level results in a rise in basal body temperature (taken when the body is at complete rest). If you take your temperature every morning upon awakening, you will note an increase of a half to a full degree within 24 to 48 hours following ovulation and this elevation will be sustained until just before your next menstrual period.

At mid-cycle, coinciding with the rupture of an egg from the ovary, approximately 25 percent of women experience some physical discomfort, a phenomenon called *Mittelschmerz*. The sensation ranges from mild, brief twinges in the lower abdomen to severe, lingering pain, sometimes accompanied by slight bleeding.

Regardless of the length or regularity of a cycle, the timing of ovulation is fairly consistent and generally predicts when menstruation will next occur. Thus, in a 35-day-long cycle, ovulation probably takes place around the 21st day; in a shorter 21-day cycle, it is likely to occur on about day 7—in each case, roughly 14 days before the onset of the next menstrual flow. (You can determine when ovulation *last* occurred simply by counting back about 14 days from the start of your very next period.)

Intense physical activity or inadequate nutrition—the result of chronic dieting, poor eating habits or anorexia—can delay or inhibit menstruation, including the very first period. Apparently, a critical ratio of fat to lean muscle tissue is necessary to activate the hypothalamus. If the level of fat is below 17 per cent of an adolescent girl's total body weight, she may not be able to menstruate. (However, there are a number of exceptions to this rule.) Oddly enough, obesity or an excess of fat can have a

14

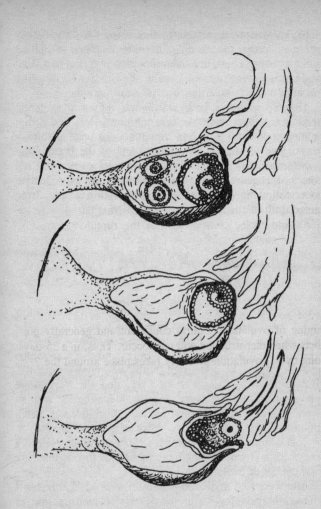

Occasionally, mild pain may accompany ovulation just as the egg is released from its follicle.

similarly disruptive effect. In this case, the fatty tissues serve to increase the amount of available estrogen—resulting in an abnormal hormone balance which prevents ovulation and normal menstruation. (Again, see Chapter III for more on menstrual irregularities or "problem periods.")

Keep in mind that the hypothalamus is the control center for thirst, hunger, appetite, sex, emotions, sleep and stress, among a variety of drives and functions, and is highly responsive to signals from other parts of the brain. That means an erratic or interrupted menstrual cycle does not necessarily point to anything amiss in the reproductive system, but may originate elsewhere—for example, from prolonged emotional distress or a chronic eating or sleeping disorder.

MENSTRUATION: ATTITUDES OLD AND NEW

During ancient times, attitudes about menstruation alternated between repulsion and exaltation. The monthly flow was called a woman's friend in those early tongues and the bleeding, self-healing process was revered as an awesome event, intimately connected with the renewal of life. However, many later societies regarded the very same phenomenon with fear and disgust. Menstruating women were sequestered from men for days, forbidden to touch plants or crops, viewed as a source of evil and disease.

In the famous words of Rome's Pliny the Elder, "Hardly can there be found a thing more monstrous than is that flux and course of theirs."

The legacy of myth and malady lingers still, although I think relatively few of us today refer to menstruation as "the curse." Happily, after centuries of neglect, medical science has finally acknowledged that pain and premenstrual mood swings are based on real physiological changes over the course of a cycle—not on emotional instability or sexual maladjustment, as was once believed.

16

According to Elizabeth Rodgers, a magazine columnist and a recognized authority on sexual behavior who has worked with William Masters and Virginia Johnson, the new enlightened and long-overdue focus on developing remedies for menstrual distress is an undeniably welcome breakthrough. However, she rightly cautions against "a scientific emphasis on the negative" rather than on the positive, life-enhancing aspects of menstruation. The latter simply don't make sensational headlines and most women give them surprisingly little, if any, thought.

Thus, few people talk about the creative energy, power, confidence and well-being that suffuse many women at the time of ovulation; the heightened senses of smell, sight and hearing; the surge of sexual excitement. When menstruation makes news, it is invariably about pain and suffering, erratic or violent swings of mood and new medical solutions to the monthly "problem."

On the other hand, some women prefer to avoid the topic altogether, fearful that any discussion of menstruation will only point up biological differences between the sexes, possibly sparking a new disenchantment with women or arousing old male fears about female instability and the onslaught of "raging hormones."

So there is either too little news or too much of the wrong kind. As Rodgers advises, "It's time to pay attention to *what we actually experience* (both good and ill) rather than accepting what society has subtly told us we should feel, whether embarrassment, depression and pain as in the past, or 'perfect health' as in the 1980s."

While menstrual distress stems from primarily physical problems, there is little doubt that regarding the cycle with dread, disgust or embarrassment can only augment any bodily-based complaint. On the other hand, false stoicism, a determination to act as if menstruation didn't exist and to ignore or resist cyclical changes, can be equally self-defeating, Rodgers sensibly argues.

The inescapable link between body and mind makes the

17

menstrual cycle inevitably both a physiological and psychological event. It is the source of internal rhythms—physical, emotional, sexual—which should be fully acknowledged, not denied or suppressed or else overplayed, out of proportion to their impact on our behavior.

If we are especially energetic at ovulation, just the opposite may occur for some of us, some of the time, as hormone levels drop and metabolic irregularities are more likely before menstruation. The frequent result of this chemical shift is a general slowing down, a heightened sensitivity and greater introspection, the need for more rest to recharge waning energies. It might well be considered an opportunity for reflection and renewal programmed right into our basic biological structure. Men are not so fortunate.

Of course, this possible premenstrual slowing of responses and flagging of energies has often been labeled in negative terms—as depression—and we have even blamed ourselves for the decline. But simply knowing the reasons for such changes and being prepared may make them far easier to manage, if not an outright advantage at certain times.

Awareness of our monthly changes can also set our mind and moods in favor of, rather than against, menstruation, as Rodgers suggests, so that we come to regard it as a kind of "sensual experience, in the same league as breast-feeding and natural childbirth." Along with such positive attitudes, simply observing the cardinal rules of well-being—rest, relaxation, adequate exercise, sensible eating—and resorting to safe, effective remedies for possible pain and discomfort can help ensure a "lifetime" of healthy, trouble-free cycles.

OLD WIVES' TALES AND MYTHS

Many ancient taboos and tales—born of the awe or fear with which men often regarded menstruating women (how could they bleed so profusely and still survive?)—are at the heart of many myths and prejudices still with us today. The following are among the most prevalent and persistent. None of them, happily, has any basis in fact.

•*Menstruation is a sign of uncleanliness and less-than-perfect health; therefore, a woman's touch during this time is undesirable and should be avoided.* In the ancient past, this myth was firmly rooted—menstruating women were believed capable of spoiling food and crops as well as bringing bad luck to hunters. As recently as the 1800s, this notion was prevalent in the Orient, where women were not permitted to work in the opium industry because it was thought that the drug would turn bitter in the presence of menstrual blood.

•*Avoid exercising during your period.* On the contrary, working out is very beneficial and women athletes generally report fewer complaints of cramping than their sedentary counterparts. By stimulating the circulatory system, physical activity helps ease muscle tensions and congested pelvic blood vessels.

•*You should not swim while you are menstruating.* False! Of course, regardless of the time of the month, swimming in very cold water may bring on muscle spasms and cramps in *any* part of the body.

•*Having intercourse during menstruation is dangerous to a woman's (or man's) health.* Of course not. A woman might experience a slight increase in susceptibility to infection anywhere in the body during this time; otherwise sex while menstruating has no ill effect on health, and orgasm may even temporarily relieve mild dysmenorrhea by accelerating menstrual flow and dispelling tensions. Surprisingly, some Europeans believe that men may be more likely to contract gonorrhea or other sex-related diseases if they have intercourse with a menstruating woman. There is *no* medical basis for this notion!

•*Women are not interested in sex or easily aroused before or during their periods*. In fact, many women report a heightened libido at this time. And instead of being offended by the aesthetics of menstruation, some women and men actually find it sexually arousing.

•*Don't eat cold foods while menstruating*. Hot foods may *feel* better when you're generally tense or experiencing menstrual twinges—but that's the only advantage. Just eat sensibly, as always.

•*Women are physically vulnerable during their periods and should curb their regular activities*. This fanciful notion may be traced back to the days when women were isolated while menstruating (sometimes in special "huts" designed for this purpose) because they were considered ill and incapacitated. But a positive attitude and participation-as-usual in daily activities are instrumental to feeling your best any time of the month.

•*Permanent waves won't take—and neither will dental fillings—while you're menstruating*. This nonsense speaks for itself—menstruation as magic or "curse."

•*Don't water plants while you're having your period*. (Or else they will wilt.) Alas, a 20th-century idea, not far removed from Pliny the Elder's injunction about Roman crops!

Notes Chapter One:

1 *Mega-Nutrition for Women*, by Richard Kunin, M.D., (McGraw-Hill,) p. 63

2 "We are only beginning to trace the paths of our instincts," observes Dr. Avodah Offit in her eloquently written book, *Night Thoughts: Reflections of a Sex Therapist*. (Congdon &

Lattes, Inc.) "As we grow older in evolution, we seem to learn more about our primitive selves—how we are governed by factors beyond our control."

3 *Women: A Book for Men* Produced by James Wagenvoord and Peyton Bailey (Avon, 1979), p. 85

4 Ibid. p. 86

Chapter 2

DYSMENORRHEA: NEW FINDINGS ABOUT MENSTRUAL PAIN

Michelle came into my office one day after battling with severe cramps on and off for about seven years—she'd finally decided she had had enough! They first started when she was about 14 and the pain was wrenching, but she never thought of doing much about it.

"I suffered mostly in silence," she admits. "On rare occasions I resorted to bed rest and a hot water bottle. Or my mother gave me some vodka or brandy, and that would bring a little relief. Of course, my friends and I talked about our periods and how much trouble they were—but we just assumed that cramps were an inevitable part of the package, the price you paid for growing up and becoming a woman."

The pain was particularly disabling during college, she recalls. "In high school my schedule was so busy and full that I often didn't have that much time to think about my cramps. But in college, I had plenty of hours between classes to dwell on my physical discomfort! Besides, the pain, always very gripping, seemed to get worse as I grew older."

Unfortunately, Michelle's cycle happens to be shorter than average and very regular: She invariably gets her period every 15 to 17 days, which means that she goes through her ordeal roughly *twice* each month. ("At a frequency of once a month I might find it twice as tolerable!'' she quips.) As if this weren't enough, her periods typically last six or seven days, making them longer than average; the bleeding is also substantial and the menstrual distress often lingers throughout.

A 30-year-old friend of mine has had painful cramps ever since she was 16, though, unlike Michelle's, hers seem to be a bit less intense than they were before. She feels a predictable array of premenstrual pangs—swelling in the breasts, aching legs, low back pain, fatigue and acne breakouts, followed by the *coup de grace*—sharp, searing pains in the lower abdomen just as her period begins. This sequence is almost always accompanied by dizziness, nausea and vomiting.

"Usually the 'attack' comes very abruptly, with hardly any warning,'' she says. "I remember being right in the middle of a final exam once when I suddenly felt violently nauseous and had to rush out of the room. My teacher must have thought I was crazy (or that I was having some sort of delayed panic attack) but at that point I didn't care about failing a test! All I knew was that I felt overwhelmingly sick and that I had just gotten my period.''

Another time she fell ill while working in a hospital lab (of all places). Her boss was outraged at first by her sudden disappearance—so she had some face-to-face explaining to do. Just two months ago, she took a new job as an administrative assistant with a well-known magazine—and she's worried about her future since she's already had to call in sick several days because of her period.

How has my long-suffering friend found relief? "When I first started visiting doctors for cramps they would prescribe powerful analgesics like Darvon. But these only numbed the pain slightly, if at all, and succeeded in knocking me out a few hours later. (One time I wound up walking around school stoned and giddy, as if I were high on marijuana!) When the effects wore off, I'd be left with a throbbing headache and a hangover, leaving me sicker than before. And once a doctor told me I was 'overreacting'

24

to my period and should take it more in stride. He suggested the pain was mostly imagined.''

But, as for happy endings: Recently, she's not only found a more understanding physician, but also a medication that eases her distress considerably and allows her to remain alert and active as well.

Menstruation and pain: For over half of all women of childbearing age, the two are chronically connected. And more than 10 percent of us are routinely incapacitated at the start of each new cycle. (Menstrual distress is reportedly the number one cause of female absenteeism from school and work.) When the problem is troublesome enough to warrant medical relief, doctors refer to it as *dysmenorrhea,* a word of Greek origin meaning difficult monthly flow.

Until quite recently, women with severe discomfort either gritted their teeth and endured it or else visited their doctors for powerful prescription painkillers—which only masked the symptoms and often drugged the patient into oblivion. Since medical science could find no biological basis for monthly pain, some physicians tended to dismiss it as primarily psychosomatic, an ''all in your head'' type of complaint.

But research during the last several years has finally pinpointed the agents responsible for about 80 percent of painful periods: Called *prostaglandins* (PGs), these incredibly potent, swift-acting, hormone-like chemicals are produced by almost every cell in the body from the brain to the lower extremities. Prostaglandins control an endless array of vital functions but unlike the wandering hormones they are strictly local messengers, influencing only the part of the body where they are made. (Among their roles are the regulation of blood clotting, the contraction of blood vessels and smooth muscles, intestinal movement, heartbeat and breathing.)

While most prostaglandins act as natural wonder drugs, some types, especially in excessive amounts, are actually internal troublemakers. For example, one group of PGs promotes the pain, swelling and inflammation that characterize arthritis. Another constricts the walls of blood vessels near the heart to trigger the crushing chest pains of angina. Still another, secreted by the lining of the uterus (endometrium), causes its smooth-muscle tissue to contract, giving rise to the spasms that accompany menstruation.

Occasionally, intense cramping, possibly with abnormal bleeding, may be the result of *secondary dysmenorrhea*, painful periods resulting from a specific organic disorder such as endometriosis, fibroid tumors, pelvic inflammatory disease, malignancy or even an IUD, among other conditions. In this case, the doctor must isolate the source of the pain before prescribing appropriate treatment. Interestingly, prostaglandins may even be involved in this type of dysmenorrhea. For more details, see p. 38.

At normal levels, prostaglandins are necessary to help the uterus shed the rich, spongy lining or endometrium it no longer needs if pregnancy does not occur. After ovulation, at the midpoint of the monthly cycle, prostaglandins are held in check by high concentrations of the hormone progesterone. The latter helps thicken the walls of the uterus with nourishing glandular tissue to create the proper haven for a fertilized egg. By the end of the cycle, however, if fertilization has not taken place, progesterone levels drop off sharply and prostaglandins rise dramatically, causing the uterus to contract and slough off its now superfluous lining.

Researchers W.Y. Chan and M. Yusoff Dawood of the Cornell University Medical College in New York City have found that women with persistently painful periods have about two to three times the level of prostaglandins in their menstrual fluid as women who are essentially symptom-free. These high concentrations produce more frequent, powerful and longer-lasting contractions, along with higher pressures within the uterus—which are experienced as spasmodic, labor-like pain. The discomfort often radiates to the back and along the thighs and legs as well.

As the walls of the uterus contract with force, blood

26

vessels are tightly squeezed, reducing circulation to hard-working muscles. The resulting loss of oxygen (and pressure buildup) also contributes to the cramping sensation. In addition, prostaglandins and related substances act directly on local nerve endings, making them more sensitive to pain. Elsewhere, an oversupply of the same kinds of prostaglandins stimulates vigorous muscle contractions within the stomach, intestines, bladder, blood vessels and other areas. This accounts for the cluster of complaints often surrounding dysmenorrhea—the nausea, vomiting, diarrhea, fatigue, frequent urination, headache and dizziness; the raw, tender feeling in nerve-rich genital tissues.

For every woman, prostaglandin levels automatically increase just before menstruation begins; apparently, it's the excessive rise that leads to painful results. Still another possible contributor to menstrual distress is a tightness or narrowing of the cervical opening from the uterus to the vagina. A narrow cervix may distend the uterus above it and delay the release of menstrual flow, giving rise to uncomfortable pressure and a prolonged or increased absorption of prostaglandins. This is probably why, for about one-third of women with dysmenorrhea, the birth of a first child—which relaxes and widens the cervix—often signals an end to troublesome cramps.

Some dysmenorrheic women are also believed to have lower-than-average blood levels of a chemical called oxytocin and normal amounts of a related substance, vasopressin, both considered uterine stimulants. According to studies, when oxytocin is low, the spasms induced primarily by vasopressin are painful and erratic. This finding simply reinforces the point that monthly cramps spring from very specific physical causes.

In fact, dysmenorrhea from a purely emotional source is very rare in clinical practice. Acute discomfort can certainly color your feelings regarding menstruation, but the physical distress comes first—attitude is *not* to blame. Of course, body and mind are so intimately connected that any chronic dread or fear of pain will probably aggravate the existing problem; it cannot possibly help. Women who suffer repeatedly without seeking a doctor's care may experience anxiety, tension, depression, emotional withdrawal and a sense of powerlessness with the onset of each monthly cycle. Such attitudes can permeate their personality and render their pain less endurable.

As Elizabeth Rodgers observes, two realities are at work: "One is the actual biochemistry of the menstrual cycle that produces so many measurable changes in a woman's body each month; and the second is the state of mind in which that biochemistry is experienced. Each reality influences the other . . . Tensing the mind and the emotions against the menstrual experience, however unknowingly, makes the experience worse. And tensing the body against menstrual pain makes the pain worse." The latter principle is recognized in childbirth, as women learn proper breathing and relaxation techniques to keep from straining the body and resisting labor pains, which will only make them more intense.

Even when severe and lingering, the pain of dysmenorrhea rarely lasts beyond one to three days into the period. Why: The mischief-making prostaglandins are released from the body along with the menstrual flow and so are greatly reduced in number after the first several days of bleeding. If, however, the flow starts out very light for the first few days, followed by heavier bleeding, the worst discomfort may be felt midway through and toward the end of the period.

Though scientists aren't fully certain why, dysmenorrhea does not generally occur in the absence of ovulation. The probable reason is that without the stimulus of progesterone, the uterine lining does not thicken as substantially, so the resulting flow is thinner and fewer prostaglandins are secreted. This explains why adolescent girls do not experience severe cramping when they first start to menstruate and up to several years after—until their cycles have become more regular and they consistently ovulate. It also accounts for why the birth control pill has often been such an effective, if indirect, remedy for dysmenorrhea. The Pill's synthetic hormones suppress natural ovulation and produce a thinner monthly flow: Again, fewer prostaglandins are released in the process, minimizing pain. In fact, scientists have confirmed that the prostaglandin content is significantly lower in the menstrual fluid of women using oral contraceptives as compared to other women.

While prescribing the Pill for painful periods was once considered a drastic regimen, the most recent verdict is that for a majority of women, especially those under 35, oral contraceptives are far safer than previously believed, and in some cases may even be outright beneficial. For example, a recent study cited in *The New England Journal of Medicine* compared the impact of differently formulated birth control pills on cholesterol, triglyceride and lipoprotein levels in the blood. The HDL or "good" cholesterol, which carries away deposits from arterial walls, tended to be highest, and LDL or undesirable cholesterol, concentrations lowest, in women using estrogen-dominant preparations. Just the reverse was true for those on relatively high progestin (synthetic progesterone) pills. The *kind* of progestin used in the different types of pills seems to play an even more significant role in the effect on blood levels of HDL.

This suggests that for at least one major risk factor in coronary disease, certain types of oral contraceptives, namely those with a relatively high ratio of estrogen to progestin, and those containing the right kind of progestin (for example, Ortho Novum) may actually have a protective effect. On the basis of this study, the researchers conclude, physicians should use caution when prescribing progestin-dominant pills for women with a known susceptibility to cardiovascular disease. For more on the Pill and who should or should not be taking it, see Chapter 7.

For one of my young patients, who complained of both unusually frequent cycles and persistent dysmenorrhea, I prescribed the birth control pill after I determined, of course, that she was seeking a reliable contraceptive as well as relief for her painful symptoms. At first she actually felt worse because the dosage of estrogen in her formula was a little too low; this artifically induced hormone imbalance caused her to start bleeding profusely, painfully and continuously for about 14 days. But when the formula was readjusted, the Pill suppressed ovulation, which diminished the number of pain-generating prostaglandins secreted by the lining of her uterus. Also, since she has been on the Pill, she has been bleeding every 25 to 28 days (rather than every 17), far closer to the timing of the average menstrual cycle.

"While the Pill is definitely not a cure-all for monthly pain—I still feel spasms once in a while—it has curbed the discomfort considerably. I am also taking a prescription medication which *directly* inhibits the release of prostaglandins (see below). Although my cramps have not dissipated completely, they are more subdued, less frequent and far more manageable," she reports.

THE NEW WONDER DRUGS?

Knowing precisely what triggers menstrual cramps has led medical science to develop a safe, specific and highly effective treatment—a class of non-steroidal, anti-inflammatory drugs (NSAIDS) that can thwart the guilty prostaglandins at their source, and thus prevent or minimize the pain. These include both over-the-counter and prescription-only remedies.

For many women, if not most, menstrual distress is confined to relatively mild, intermittent cramps which subside after a day or two and do not disrupt normal activities. In this case, relief can be obtained from proper exercise and diet, heating pads, warm, relaxing baths and other natural measures, along with over-the-counter preparations if necessary, such as the familiar, long-standing remedy Midol, which can ease painful twinges and abdominal bloating.

Midol works by gently inhibiting the release of certain prostaglandins that promote muscle contraction and inflammation within the uterine lining and elsewhere. It may also relieve mild-to-moderate discomfort by relaxing the muscles of the pelvis and gastrointestinal tract. As an antiprostaglandin, it may act, too, as an anticoagulant or blood-thinning drug—and so may keep the menstrual flow from forming potentially painful clots. The active ingredient in most other store-bought menstrual remedies such as Pamprin is *acetaminophen* which may effectively curb pain but does not counteract inflammation or the release of prostaglandins. (Since some prostaglandins are secreted before the visible flow, Midol may be most beneficial if taken about one day before the expected period. Pamprin and other acetaminophen-based products do not prevent pain from starting and so should be taken only to relieve distress.)

For more severe pain, other prostaglandin inhibitors are available by prescription only, marketed under such names as Motrin, Ponstel, Naprosyn, Anaprox and Indocin. The corresponding generic names for these are, respectively, ibuprofen, flufenamic or mefenamic acid, naproxen, naproxen sodium and indomethacin. Such medications were originally developed for the relief of arthritic pain (also a prostaglandin-induced disorder) and have recently been approved by the FDA for use against menstrual cramps as well.

Properly given, such drugs restrict or block the synthesis of prostaglandins by the cells of the uterine lining where they originate. As a result, they reduce the pressures within the uterus along with the force and frequency of its labor-like contractions. These compounds also counteract prostaglandins already present and decrease the volume of menstrual flow, which in itself may help account for the pain relief. As mentioned earlier, fewer prostaglandins are released when periods are relatively light and short.

While they all work against the "bad" prostaglandins, each compound has a different mode of action, so if one preparation does not provide marked relief, you may have better results with another. The *cost* of any drug therapy should definitely be considered in addition to how well it works: Obviously, over-the-counter prostaglandin inhibitors are the most economical choice if they work for you. For example, 60 tablets of Midol cost $3.96 and 100 tablets sells for $6.60. Since Motrin is the least expensive prescription medication in the lineup (costing about $29.75 per 100 as compared to $57.25 for Naprosyn; both generics, of course, would be considerably cheaper), I would definitely recommend trying it *first*. Most of my patients with dysmenorrhea have found it highly effective.

Though the success rate for antiprostaglandins is very impressive—relief is good to excellent for 65 to 100 percent of patients—don't expect overnight results. Often my patients must take a selected drug for several days during at least *two* menstrual cycles before we can determine whether or not the remedy controls their pain effectively or if the dosage is just right. Fortunately, these preparations minimize or eliminate distress without causing dizziness or fatigue or altering moods; they do not interfere with productivity at work or home. As such, they can help women meet their goal of staying fit, functional and symptom-free throughout their periods without having to resort to mind-numbing, habit-forming, expensive narcotics. Happily, even women whose complaints are not completely curbed by such remedies require less use of painkillers and suffer fewer hours of disabling pain.

In the past, and for severe cases, physicians recommended that women take Motrin and related compounds at least two days before the expected onset of menstrual bleeding to help stamp out all traces of prostaglandins before they could be produced in any significant amounts. But current thinking now suggests that this all-out, in-advance approach with prescription drugs is not necessary since prostaglandins are rapidly produced and excreted; not stored in the body for any length of time.

Taking the drugs after your period begins and not before also rules out the possibility that you may be pregnant while on the medication. So far, there is no documented evidence that these remedies are teratogenic (harmful to a developing fetus) when used to treat dysmenorrhea or more severe ailments. For example, women who must rely on antiprostaglandins continually and at higher doses for such diseases as rheumatoid arthritis or lupus have not been shown to have a significantly greater risk of bearing children with birth defects than the normal population. However, it's generally best to avoid *any* unnecessary drug during pregnancy.

One of the two known possible risks associated with antiprostaglandins and pregnancy is premature closure of the *patent ductus* in the heart of a developing embryo— certainly not relevant to women with dysmenorrhea. The drugs can also postpone labor since they curb the smooth-muscle contractions of the uterine wall which normally help expel the fully developed fetus.

To sum up, the present-day consensus is that a woman should wait for the first signs of either cramping or bleeding before taking any prescription antiprostaglandin. The important *exception* to this rule may be during the *initial* therapeutic trial period when a physician and patient are trying to determine whether a certain medication is an appropriate and successful treatment. Mindful of the minimal potential risks, a patient and I may agree to try out a particular drug for two successive months by starting it shortly before menstruation. With this strategy, we take every precaution to ensure the maximum effectiveness of the drug, so that if a patient does *not* respond well, we cannot blame it on either procedure or timing. (Based on the results of the "trial," we aim to establish a dose that will be effective and safe when taken during subsequent cycles, just at the start of a period.)

Before beginning *any* therapy always tell your doctor

about other medications you are taking or any allergies you have which might interfere with or contraindicate your treatment. For example, aspirin should not be combined with the prescription antiprostaglandins.

Happily, the side effects of prostaglandin inhibitors and antagonists are relatively mild and usually reported to be tolerable. The main reason for this is that you don't have to stay on these powerful drugs for generally more than two to four days each month. If you were taking the very same medication for arthritis you would need a considerably higher round-the-clock dosage every day, of course, which is why any drug-related complications are more likely to be linked to arthritic patients, not to women with dysmenorrhea.

Motrin (ibuprofen) should not be prescribed for women who have aspirin-induced allergies, ulcers, gastritis or nasal polyps. The same caution applies to those who are hypersensitive to the drug itself (signalled by severe rash and/or breathing difficulties). Other reported side effects include dizziness, water retention and edema. So far, animal studies, involving dosages of up to 1,600 mgs. a day, have not revealed any evidence that the drug is teratogenic.

The adverse reactions to flufenamic and mefenamic acid (and other compounds in the fenamate family) range from nausea, digestive discomfort and diarrhea to severe anemia, dizziness, drowsiness, nervousness, headache, blurry vision, rash and mild toxicity of the kidneys or liver. In rats, mefanamic acid impairs fertility, and its safety during early pregnancy has not yet been determined.

Indomethacin is probably one of the most potent of the prescription drugs—though, as with the others, possible complications are mostly dose-related and often disappear completely when the intake is reduced. Potential complaints include severe headache or gastrointestinal distress, rash, blurred vision, corneal and retinal disturbances and certain forms of anemia.

34

Since the prostaglandins that trigger cramps have a localized effect, scientists reason that drugs designed to suppress them can work even more powerfully and with fewer side effects if they are taken in the form of vaginal or rectal suppositories or intrauterine devices coated with an antiprostaglandin formula. Since they would be quickly absorbed by neighboring tissues, these drugs could permeate the sexual organs in higher concentrations than if they were taken by mouth and ultimately dispersed throughout the bloodstream. This would make systemic side effects less likely, yet deliver a stronger dose right where it was needed. For example, like the Pill, IUDs treated with any one of the prostaglandin inhibitors would be ideal for women with dysmenorrhea who also wanted reliable contraception. Scientists are currently investigating the effectiveness of *progesterone*-saturated IUDs (marketed as Progestasert). Progesterone has been shown to slow down uterine contractions in laboratory animals and the contraceptive device containing the hormone is being studied to determine its usefulness against dysmenorrhea.

BASIC REMEDIES

While antiprostaglandins or the Pill can offer dramatic relief for the most stubborn cases of dysmenorrhea, by and large the best approach is to start with the mildest, most conservative measures first. At the very least, they can be beneficial adjuncts to any course of drug therapy, should it be required. A number of simpler remedies may work some minor miracles or make you feel more relaxed and comfortable when menstrual distress is at its peak:

•*Heat:* Whether you prefer hot water bottles, towels, heating pads, saunas or steambaths, heat applied to the abdominal area will help ease muscle spasms, dilate congested blood vessels and simply feel good. Warm showers or leisurely baths will relax the body's tensed-up muscles overall and have a mentally calming effect. Hot soups and teas can also bring some relief.

•*Massage:* The "laying on of hands" over stomach, abdomen and back is another natural muscle relaxant and circulation stimulant, especially when done with soothing, deep-heating ointments or creams.

•*Exercise:* Stretching and limbering routines can unlock clenched muscles: It's already known that a relaxed muscle, whether within the uterus or anywhere else, will simply hurt less than one that is taut and rigid. A regimen that strengthens both the abdomen and back will make you less susceptible to menstrual backaches. And the improved blood flow that follows any regular workout may help rid the body of extra fluid. Sustained *aerobic* exercise such as swimming or jogging enhances endurance and has a naturally tranquilizing, mood-elevating effect.

•*Breathing:* Learning to breathe deeply and rhythmically can transport much-needed oxygen throughout the body, enabling muscles to stay loose and relaxed. Remember, breathing exercises are the basis of the Lamaze technique to ease childbirth pain, a principle that may help make menstruation more endurable.

•*Sex & Orgasm:* Sexual intercourse is a natural tension reliever, and some women report fewer cramps and less low back pain after orgasm. This is probably the result of the dilation of congested pelvic blood vessels. Following orgasm, there may be a temporary increase in the rate of menstrual flow—which will help expel the pain-producing prostaglandins that much sooner.

•*Diet:* Eating a wide variety of foods with ample fiber will keep bowels loose and prevent constipation which can aggravate menstrual symptoms. Light fare—fresh fruits and vegetables, a moderate amount of cereal grains, low-fat dairy products, fish and poultry—is most beneficial. There is some good evidence that calcium supplements can help relieve cramps in a number of women. Salt intake should also be reduced to minimize bloating.

•*Alcohol:* A 3-ounce glass of wine or a liquor-laced hot drink mildly counteracts the release of uterine-contracting prostaglandins and subdues the central nervous system: The effect is to quiet spasms temporarily, elevate mood and heighten your tolerance to pain. Alcohol is also a strong vasodilator, opening up constricted vessels for easier circulation.

•*Childbirth:* As already mentioned, following delivery of their first child, many women actually experience pain-free periods for the first time in their lives.

•*Weight Loss:* Obesity can aggravate menstrual pain because the body's fatty tissues produce extra estrogen which spurs the growth of the uterine lining and often results in a heavier monthly flow. This added hormonal stimulus may boost the level of prostaglandins issued by the uterus, giving rise to greater discomfort. So keeping weight down is yet another way to put a limit on the undesirable prostaglandins.

•*Clothing:* Avoid binding, tight-fitting pantyhose, panty girdles and jeans which can hamper circulation and intensify abdominal discomfort.

•*Analgesics:* Over-the-counter pain relievers such as aspirin, Tylenol, Datril and Excedrin may be effective against the "garden" variety of cramps. Other women respond well to Midol, Pamprin, Vanquish, Cope and similar preparations marketed for menstrual distress. For example, Midol combines an analgesic and prostaglandin inhibitor with an antispasmodic ingredient. It also has a mild diuretic effect which helps rid the body of excess water.

•*Electricity:* Some women have reported considerable relief from small machines called "TENS" (transcutaneous electrical nerve stimulators). Available from and monitored by physicians, these devices trigger tiny amounts of electric current that are apparently able to "jam" a variety of pain signals—including the ones for menstruation.

SECONDARY DYSMENORRHEA

So far this chapter has highlighted the causes and remedies of primary dysmenorrhea—painful periods occurring in the absence of organic disease or any underlying complications. But while less common, and generally occurring later in life, secondary dysmenorrhea may herald a number of disorders such as endometriosis (nicknamed "the working woman's disease"), polyps, fibroids and even result from an IUD.

Some recent research suggests that an overabundance of prostaglandins may play a role in cases of secondary dysmenorrhea. When an organ is inflamed, it generally releases a higher-than-normal level of prostaglandins. Sure enough, investigators have discovered such an increase in the uterine linings of women with endometriosis, fibroids and other conditions. The uterine "trauma" or white blood cell "pooling" caused by insertion of an IUD stimulates prostaglandin output, which could account for both the heavier flow and more intense cramping often reported by wearers of the contraceptive device. For this reason, women with IUDs who suffer from unusually painful or heavy periods often find tremendous relief from antiprostaglandin therapy. The drugs that have been especially effective are flufenamic acid, ibuprofen and naproxen.

In rare cases, secondary dysmenorrhea may stem from a congenital abnormality such as cervical obstruction or an unperforated hymen. As a result, the uterus becomes distended and menstrual fluid may not exit easily or at all, leading to a prolonged absorption of prostaglandins. Women born with such structural irregularities, correctible through minor surgery, generally experience the resulting dysmenorrhea as adolescents, usually from the time of their very first menstrual cycle. (All other types of secondary dysmenorrhea usually surface later in life, which is one possible way to distinguish it from the primary kind.)

Endometriosis: This is the most prevalent of the reasons for secondary dysmenorrhea—suffered by one third of those complaining of pelvic pain or infertility—and its incidence appears to be increasing. Unfortunately, it may progress insidiously and remain undetected because it is readily confused with just-plain menstrual cramps. Women who have been conditioned to endure disabling monthly discomfort may simply brace themselves for the worst and fail to seek a physician's help, even in the face of severe and unusual distress.

The spasms often triggered by endometriosis begin well before and continue for a significant time after the onset of regular menstrual bleeding; the disease may also be marked by painful intercourse, rectal pressure or persistent pelvic soreness. Sometimes, however, it is virtually painless and asymptomatic. How endometriosis develops: Tissue much like that lining the uterus takes root and grows prolifically on the surface of other neighboring internal organs, such as the ovaries, intestines, bladder and Fallopian tubes. Like the normal endometrium, these spongy growths thicken and disintegrate with the hormonal fluctuations of the monthly cycle. But unlike menstrual fluid, these sloughed-off cells have no natural outlet so the body tries to absorb them. The result may be cysts, scarring, inflammation, adhesions and possible permanent damage to the affected areas.

The same surge of hormones that prompts the buildup of normal uterine tissue stimulates the misplaced endometrium as well. This is why the disease flares up around the time of menstruation and so often masquerades as a painful period. But if the cramps are intense, persistent and unresponsive to antiprostaglandin or contraceptive therapy, endometriosis should be suspected.

Endometriosis is believed to have a strong genetic component because those with a family history are especially susceptible. (One-third of women with a severe case of the disease are likely to have a close relative who was similarly afflicted.) It has been dubbed the "working women's disease" because there is some not clearly understood connection between delayed childbearing and increased risk of developing endometriosis. If left untreated, the spreading endometrium can damage the ovaries and Fallopian tubes, leading to infertility. When it implants in the intestines, sharp pains resembling those of appendicitis may result.

A detailed, accurate medical history and a pelvic exam performed by a skilled physician with experienced hands who can detect growths behind the uterus are excellent diagnostic tools.

An exploratory diagnostic procedure called laparoscopy may enable the doctor to inspect the pelvic organs directly and give more accurate diagnosis. A small incision is made in the navel through which a periscope is inserted, affording an internal view. (Of course, if the endometriosis is well-camouflaged, located just behind the uterus, a physician may possibly miss it with this method, which involves a one- to two-day hospital stay.)

As for treatment: A low estrogen, high progestin birth control pill such as Ovral, Ovulin or Norlestrin given for a limited period of time may help check the development of both normal and abnormal endometrium but cannot cure the disease. Danazol, an androgen-like steroid drug (synthetic derivative of the male hormone, testosterone) gives the pelvic organs a "rest" by inducing a kind of pseudo-menopause. It stops ovulation, blocks the release of the ovary-stimulating hormones LH and FSH and so shuts down the menstrual cycle completely. Levels of estrogen and progesterone remain relatively low and hormone receptors in endometrial tissue are also suppressed, which means that even minimal amounts of circulating hormones will not stimulate any further growth of endometrial tissue. As a result, without its usual chemical support, the endometriosis starts to wither away. By bringing the menstrual cycle and the monthly revival of diseased endometrium to a temporary halt, Danazol simply allows the healing process to begin.

This powerful drug may be well-tolerated, with minor weight gain, skin oiliness and acne flareups among the leading possible complaints. However, other women experience a range of menopause-related symptoms while taking the drug, such as hot flashes, night sweats and vaginal dryness, as well as some androgenic (male hormone-related) side effects. In spite of these, Danazol is a useful drug, providing relief of symptoms for many patients.

When the disease is advanced and surgery is indicated, several weeks or months of Danazol therapy beforehand can help shrink the endometrial growths as much as possible to simplify the operation. Surgery for widespread endometriosis is a delicate, complicated, risky procedure precisely because so many vital organs may be involved. Often, the implanted tissue cannot be cut away or cauterized entirely and the condition may well recur later on. It is believed that Danazol administered *after* surgery may help prevent or minimize future outbreaks of the disease.

A medical history and manual pelvic exam, including a rectal/vaginal exam, may uncover not only endometriosis but also such problems as ovarian cysts, uterine abnormalities, IUDs and pelvic inflammatory disease, all of which can result in abnormal or persistently painful bleeding. Based on the results of this all-important manual exam, blood tests, genital cultures or pelvic sonograms may be necessary for additional diagnostic information. A D&C (dilation and curettage) may be both diagnostic and therapeutic.

In a D&C, the opening of the cervix is stretched with a series of dilating instruments. Then a small curette or spoon-like sharpened device is placed in the uterine cavity to scrape off the lining in methodical, clockwise fashion. The procedure can both detect existing disease and serve as treatment for endometrial polyps (small benign growths of the mucous membranes).

Fibroids: Ninety-nine percent of all fibroid tumors in the muscle walls of the uterus are harmless and benign, though they can be quite large, possibly resulting in pain and abnormal monthly bleeding. Your physician may decide to perform a D&C to remove the fibroids and stem the heavy flow if these growths are small and removable by the vaginal route. More likely, however, if the growths are large and intrusive enough, you may require a *myomectomy*, a procedure which involves shelling tissue mass out of the uterine wall; this may curb the excess bleeding while keeping the uterus (and your potential for childbearing) intact.

A hysterectomy or complete removal of the uterus, is a drastic, last-resort procedure which is not generally called for in the case of fibroid tumors, except under unusual circumstances, such as when their size is larger than that of a 12-week-pregnant uterus or when they are rapidly growing.

Diagnosis is usually made during a pelvic examination and can be confirmed by a sonogram (simply speaking, a device which takes pictures of your uterus by means of ultrasound waves rather than X-rays. *Note:* Since excessive or abnormal bleeding could also be a sign of cancer of the endometrium, uterus or other part of the reproductive system (most are highly curable when detected early) this possibility should definitely be ruled out, especially if you are over 40.

Chapter 3

PROBLEM PERIODS:
MENSTRUAL IRREGULARITIES

Recently, a junior colleague of mine heard I was working on a book about the menstrual cycle and started asking me a number of questions about periods that abruptly deviate from their usual, expected pattern. Why should they be suddenly lighter or shorter than normal, for example? After hearing a brief biology lecture in return for her apparent interest, she admitted that the reason for her curiosity was not a burning desire for new medical knowledge, but rather worry about her own erratic cycle, of late. After years of menstruating "normally," she had noticed a markedly scanty flow that lasted three days instead of the typical four. Her imagination started leaping wildly. "Could this be the result of a tumor?" she asked.

A patient came in not long ago with just the opposite complaint: a very heavy, steady menstrual flow after a history of "light to moderate" bleeding. She reported having gained about 25 pounds in the last six months, but otherwise described herself to be in "excellent shape." Like my friend, she wanted to know if the change in her menstrual pattern could possibly be the result of a "serious problem."

I have also treated (mostly with reassurance) young teenage girls who have not yet begun to menstruate, among them, a wiry, 14-year-old gymnastics genius and running

43

enthusiast. In her case, vigorous physical training and low body fat are the most probable reasons for the "delay."

Unusual periods—scanty, excessive, erratic or non-existent—often occur at the beginning and end of active menstruation—during early adolescence and/or in the years preceding the menopause (when the female cycle is either just getting started or winding down). However, menstrual mishaps can take place any time throughout your fertile years, for any number of reasons (mostly *not* a cause for alarm). In this chapter, we will take a look at the most common irregularities, why they happen and how to control them.

DELAYED MENARCHE

Failure to menstruate for the first time well past the age of puberty is referred to as delayed menarche or primary amenorrhea. If you have reached your teens without having a period, many explanations are possible. For example, since menstrual patterns are usually inherited, chances are if your mother or aunt started menstruating at 14 or 15, you probably will, too.

If you are underweight or have been dieting excessively, or are a serious, competitive athlete, insufficient body fat or the stress of strenuous workouts may disrupt the complex hormonal interplay necessary to activate the normal cycle. (See more on exercise, sports and menstruation later on in this chapter.) Anxiety, grief or any severe emotional trauma, along with certain drugs and diet pills may also upset the hormonal balance. However, if you have passed your sixteenth birthday without a menstrual period, it's a good idea to visit your doctor to rule out any medical disorder or physical abnormality that may be suppressing your hormone levels or obstructing the monthly flow. Of course, if you are already sexually active, you must be checked for possible pregnancy as well!

Failure to menstruate can sometimes be caused by

structural, inborn defects of the reproductive tract, such as an absent or malformed vagina, uterus or ovaries. For example, the normal hymen—the membrane separating internal and external genital organs—in a woman who has not had sexual intercourse is equipped with an opening large enough to permit the release of menstrual fluid as well as the insertion of a tampon. On rare occasions, this opening or perforation is nonexistent, so menstrual blood cannot escape. The "imperforate hymen" can be corrected by a simple surgical procedure.

Delayed menarche can also result from a faulty connection between the ovaries and brain, where the sex-gland-stimulating hormones originate. Remember, since a number of glands and organs and hormones must engage in the menstrual drama, a miscue by any one of them can upset the entire performance.

By conducting certain tests, your doctor can determine why and where the problem exists and prescribe the appropriate solution. He or she should undertake a thorough medical history, which involves questioning you about specific disorders you may have now or once had, such as diabetes, hepatitis, coronary disease, cancer, thyroid or adrenal disturbances, eating disorders (malnutrition, obesity, anorexia, bulimia), exercise routines, and, very rarely, central nervous system disorders which could be impeding menstruation. Treatment with chemotherapy or radiation can also suppress the normal cycle. In addition, the known menstrual patterns of your mother, grandmother, sisters, aunts or cousins should be considered, along with your daily eating habits, lifestyle and possible sources of stress.

During the physical/gynecological exam that follows, the doctor will note your degree of breast development and growth of pubic hair, as well as height and weight to determine if menarche is way behind schedule. (The appearance of "secondary sexual characteristics"—breasts, pubic hair, axillary or under-arm hair and a noticeable growth spurt—usually precedes the onset of the first period by about two years.) He may test you for levels of the

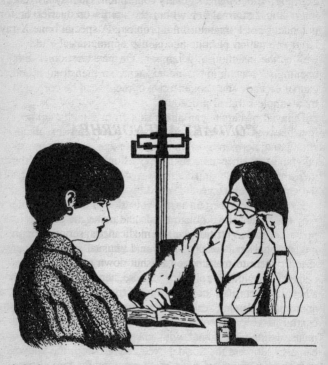

It is important to provide your doctor with a thorough medical history.

crucial hormones, estrogen, progesterone prolactin testosterone, FSH and LH if he suspects something amiss in the hypothalamus-pituitary-ovary connection. He may also check for any abnormalities within the uterus or ovaries or for evidence of a chromosomal problem. A special bone X-ray for evaluation of bone-age is also appropriate.

Quite commonly, the absence of menstruation is simply a constitutional delay. If all tests are normal, in time, spontaneous menses generally occur.

SECONDARY AMENORRHEA

Secondary amenorrhea is the cessation of periods for longer than three months in an already menstruating (non-pregnant) woman. Since the cycle depends on the perfect timing and sensitive relay of messages between ovaries and brain, any major upheaval caused by substantial weight gain or loss, chronic undernutrition, certain medications, serious diseases, emotional crisis or prolonged and unusual stress can cause the system to malfunction or shut down completely.

If your doctor has ruled out pregnancy and your pelvic exam is normal, he may conduct such procedures as a cervical mucus evaluation, hormonal analyses or an endometrial biopsy, to measure the amount of estrogen and progesterone in your body and to see whether you have ovulated. The level of a key pituitary hormone, prolactin, should be determined by a blood test. If this is elevated, he may suggest that a CT scan be performed to detect any existing tumor in the pituitary.

When asked for your medical history, be sure to report any unusual weight gain or loss and the method of contraception you have been using. In a small number of women, use of the Pill can suppress menstruation for months after being discontinued. This "post-pill amenorrhea" is almost always self-correcting or else treatable with a drug called Clomid which can activate the monthly cycle once again when you are trying to become pregnant. (If your menstrual periods were

47

normal before starting the Pill, then you will need to be evaluated completely if periods are still irregular six months after stopping the medication.)

In some cases, secondary amenorrhea is the result of a direct assault on the pituitary caused by internal bleeding or infection from a previous childbirth or trauma. Abnormalities of thyroid hormone production may also cause cessation of menses. Usually, if no organic disorder is to blame, finding and eliminating the underlying cause is treatment enough: A return to normal eating patterns, a break from rigorous physical training, the successful management of disease or stress, will be all that's necessary to restore menstrual regularity and fertility.

For women with persistent amenorrhea who have not responded to traditional measures new chemical strategies may help: Recently, scientists at the University of Essen in West Germany found that administering a nasal spray with minute amounts of luteinizing hormone (LH) to nonmenstruating women returned more than half the group to normal cycles within just a few weeks. Several of the women became pregnant within a year. Scientists in the U.S. are also investigating biochemical ways to stimulate ovulation and restore normal periods. (See below for details on currently established ways of treating amenorrhea and irregular periods.)

MENORRHAGIA—HEAVY, ERRATIC BLEEDING

As with primary and secondary amenorrhea, this phenomenon may be stress- or diet-related, or the result of some organic disorder. Generally, it is a sign of failure to ovulate due to or resulting in an inadequate release of key hormones.

A brief review of how the menstrual cycle works will help you understand why a depressed hormone level can lead to an irregular or unusually heavy flow. As you have

48

seen in Chapter 1, both estrogen and progesterone are necessary to stimulate growth of the uterine lining (endometrium) in preparation for a fertilized egg. Estrogen, secreted near the beginning of the cycle, starts the womb-building ritual and progesterone, released in substantial amounts during the second half of the cycle, continues nourishing and enriching the spongy-layered tissue. If no fertilized egg is forthcoming, however, further ovarian production of both hormones serves no purpose, so their supply dwindles sharply. Without such support, the lining breaks down soon after, a mixture of fluid, mucus, discarded cells and blood that issues forth as menstruation—the start of another new cycle.

If ovulation—the release of a ripened egg from one of the ovaries—does not occur, then no progesterone is produced, which means that the uterine lining is nourished by estrogen alone. With no cue from the rise and fall of progesterone, the endometrium may continue to develop unchecked as long as adequate estrogen is present. When the lining eventually disintegrates, it does so erratically, without the regulating influence of ovulation and the pattern of progesterone secretion and withdrawal. Aside from being unpredictable in timing, such (anovulatory) bleeding is also typically irregular in amount and duration, varying according to how much estrogen has been produced and how long it has remained at a certain level in the body.

For example, if a good number of follicles in the ovary are present and actively churning out the hormone, and if as some degenerate, new ones promptly take over, then the level of estrogen will remain high or even increase, and the endometrium may continue to grow for weeks or months. If development of the lining goes on due to a constant flow of estrogen, the endometrium will become too thick, will outgrow its blood supply and will begin to shed erratically, producing irregular and prolonged bleeding.

It is said that anovulatory cycles are rarely accompanied by cramps; however, the flow is often excessively heavy and prolonged because the endometrial layer has simply had more time to grow before being sloughed away. (Occasionally, the loss of large volumes of blood can throw someone into shock.)

Such abnormal, uninterrupted stimulation by estrogen alone may lead to severe mastalgia (breast pain) and cystic changes in the breast. Sometimes ovulation does occur, but progesterone production remains lower than necessary so cycles are still irregular, often marked by premenstrual spotting or staining.

It has already been mentioned that periods during the first two years after menarche often take place without ovulation: If menstruation is very unpredictable during this time, with light periods followed by heavy ones or long intervals without periods at all, it is not usually a cause for concern. However, if this condition lingers on into late adolescence or appears for the first time in an adult, a physician should be consulted.

Menorrhagia can occasionally signal disorders of pregnancy, such as possible miscarriage or an ectopic pregnancy. During miscarriage, the placenta, not firmly implanted in the uterine wall, may begin to slough off, often painlessly at first, issuing as a pinker, brighter flow than the usual period and culminating in severe cramping. In an ectopic pregnancy, the fertilized egg takes root outside the uterine cavity, usually lodged in a Fallopian tube. With the egg growing elsewhere in an abnormal way, hormonal production is frequently lower than in a normal pregnancy. This may cause the uterine lining to slough, producing vaginal bleeding. As the egg enlarges within the narrow tube, severe lower abdominal pain will result. This abnormally planted cluster of fetal cells can cause a life-threatening rupture if a physician does not quickly intervene.

The presence of cervicitis (inflammation of the cervix) or either uterine or cervical polyps may precipitate heavy bleeding or spotting between expected periods, especially after sexual intercourse. The same holds for tumors, IUDs or endometriosis, which is why the sudden onset of heavy, unplanned bleeding warrants a thorough checkup.

Erratic, often copious (breakthrough) bleeding may occur during the first few months of taking oral contraceptives, particularly the lower-dose pills, in which the hormone levels are not quite adequate enough to maintain a stable uterine lining but are effective in preventing ovulation. Your doctor may decide to change your prescription to another low-dose formula which frequently prevents this irregular bleeding. Once the uterus has become adjusted to the lower amounts of hormones in the pills (usually within two to three cycles) this dysfunctional bleeding disappears.

In older women, the occurrence of irregular cycles—shorter or longer than normal and often marked by heavy, prolonged bleeding—may signal the onset of the climacteric, the five- to 10-year interval of hormonal decline culminating in menopause. If you are postmenopausal and any bleeding, light or heavy, occurs six or more months after your final period, you should see your doctor who will probably advise an endometrial biopsy or D&C to check for possible signs of cancer. This is especially important if you are on estrogen replacement therapy (ERT). (See also Chapter 5.)

At any age, excess body fat can disrupt the hormone balance. It increases the synthesis of estrogen from precursors (fats are the raw material from which estrogen is made), adding to the existing supply. With too much estrogen, the menstrual cycle and ovulation may be thrown off—the reason overweight women so frequently report irregular periods as well as trouble conceiving. Thus, losing a sufficient amount of weight is often the key to restoring a regular flow.

MAKING THE DIAGNOSIS

If you are persistently irregular, your doctor may want to pinpoint the source of trouble by prescribing progesterone, most commonly Provera tablets (a synthetic form of progesterone), for about seven days. After the progesterone is discontinued, the abrupt withdrawal of the hormone should cause the lining of the uterus to break down, just as it would if the progesterone were naturally secreted by the body and then reduced. If so-called withdrawal bleeding results within four to seven days after stopping the drug, your doctor will know that enough estrogen has been produced by the ovaries to prime the uterine lining and that the cervix and vagina are normal. The body's failure to produce any or enough of its own progesterone is most likely the root of the problem.

If very little or no withdrawal bleeding occurs as a result of the short-term progesterone "test," then your ovaries may simply not be making enough estrogen to build up the endometrium, so that the artificial stimulation and withdrawal of progesterone has no marked effect. Or, this could mean that there is an abnormality in the vagina, cervix or uterus that may be interfering with menstruation.

To rule out other possibilities, your doctor might check your levels of FSH and LH, the pituitary hormones that stimulate your ovaries' follicles to secrete estrogen and progesterone. If these are too low or too high, this could point to an abnormality in the way signals are exchanged between brain and ovary. He may also look for unsuspected adrenal or thyroid disease, an ovarian or brain-based tumor or metabolic disturbances. Any one of these could suppress ovulation and thus bring about a relative shortage of progesterone in the body. He might also see whether you're producing too much androgen (male hormone), which may throw your cycle out of balance as well. Too much male hormone is often announced by an overgrowth of body hair and/or extensive acne.

Obviously, the same disorder may point to a number of

different possible causes and conditions, which is why a doctor's diagnosis is *crucial* when menstrual cycles are persistently or unaccountably irregular.

TREATMENT

If you're heavy and suffer from menorrhagia, your doctor may prescribe a change of diet before resorting to any other treatment. If low progesterone is to blame for the menstrual malfunction, which results in profuse bleeding, emergency control is possible by taking Provera. To prevent withdrawal bleeding when the progesterone is discontinued, one hormone tablet may then be given every day for 10 additional days. However, in some women, levels of estrogen are also abnormally low—so a combination of estrogen and progesterone (in the form of an oral contraceptive) would be more likely to curb or regulate bleeding. The regimen is usually continued for three to six months, depending on the patient's medical history.* Should hormone therapy prove ineffective, a D&C may be performed. (For a description of this procedure, see p. 41)

If your mother was given DES during pregnancy and you are troubled with irregular periods, your doctor should closely examine your vagina and cervix with a narrow speculum. Pap smear, palpation of pelvic organs, tissue staining, colposcopic examination and possible biopsy are also recommended. If you are over 20, a D&C may be performed to diagnose and treat any persistently erratic

---

*If you are still in your early teens and your physician is prescribing oral contraceptives, your parents may be puzzled and possibly disturbed by this apparently "precocious" treatment. But if you are flowing irregularly, your physician should explain that you need a proper balance of estrogen and progesterone for a *limited* period of time: the fact that this combination formula happens to be packaged in the form of a birth control pill may then be easier for parents to accept.

bleeding and the possible buildup of excess endometrial tissue (hyperplasia). The procedure is also used to scrape away uterine polyps, another common source of menorrhagia. When abnormal bleeding occurs during or after menopause, a D&C is done to rule out endometrial cancer; if a local overgrowth of cells is causing the problem, the operation itself will possibly cure it.

OLIGOMENORRHEA

This is a condition in which a woman menstruates only occasionally, perhaps once or twice a year. It is most often due to polycystic ovarian syndrome (PCO) or inadequate stimulation of otherwise normally developed ovaries.

PCO syndrome is characterized by increased male hormone production from ovarian and perhaps adrenal sources, as well as abnormalities in levels of FSH and LH (the hormones that stimulate the ovaries). As a result, ovulation rarely occurs. Instead, the ovaries develop multiple follicles with cyst formation which produce a constant level of estrogen and *no* progesterone. Since menstrual bleeding occurs only rarely due to this constant stimulation of the uterine lining by estrogen, there is an increase in precancerous and malignant conditions of the endometrium.

In contrast to the PCO syndrome which is characterized by constant ovarian production of estrogen, patients with inadequate secretion of the stimulatory hormones, FSH and LH and normal ovaries are frequently *hypoestrogenic* (meaning they produce abnormally *low* levels of estrogen). If the uterine lining does not receive enough estrogen to make it grow, there will be no menstrual bleeding. Stress, inadequate body weight, rigorous exercise or physical training all are common in young women and may prevent proper release of the hormones necessary to stimulate the ovaries. Oligomenorrhea may also result from birth control pill use until the cycle rights itself, as well as infection of the uterine lining or irritation by an IUD.

Oligomenorrhea is often treated with drugs which can provide the proper amounts of hormonal stimulation to the uterus, resulting in cyclical bleeding. If a woman already has enough estrogen, she may be given progesterone by Provera tablets for seven days. Then the hormone will be discontinued, which induces withdrawal uterine bleeding a few days later.

Because it elevates the body's estrogen, and depresses progesterone, polycystic ovarian syndrome may entail a slightly higher risk of breast cancer if left untreated.

EXERCISE, SPORTS AND MENSTRUAL IRREGULARITY

In California, women who want to enter professional boxing matches have had to certify that they will not be competing during a period (to the best of their knowledge). Promising junior athletes of 14 or 15 have been barred from scholastic competition in swimming and track events if they have not yet begun to menstruate. And at one girls' school, students are required to miss gym classes during the first one or two days of their period—in order not to "interfere with fertility," as the director has maintained.

A 30-year-old woman, recently married, has been running more than 30 miles a week and is now menstruating irregularly. Every time she skips her expected period, she worries that she might be pregnant. Her companion, however, has stopped menstruating altogether and wonders whether she will ever be able to conceive.

Are any of these concerns or restrictions justified? Or are they based on groundless fears and myths?

With record numbers of women now participating in sports, medical (and media) attention has turned to the impact of vigorous exercise on the female reproductive system. Happily, some of the earliest alarms and reservations have turned out to be false: For example, beliefs that pelvic organs would drop or severely loosen as a result of distance running have been completely reversed, since studies show that such sustained conditioning actually tones and supports the reproductive region and strengthens the muscles that hold it together. And women athletes report fewer complaints of cramps and bloating before or during a period. One possible reason: Working up a good sweat during invigorating aerobic exercise acts as a natural diuretic, easing salt and water retention. Physical activity also spurs the release of endorphins, the body's natural mood-boosting, morphine-like chemicals.

However, some effects of sports and exercise include an apparent (though so far benign and reversible) alteration or temporary shutdown of the menstrual cycle. About 10 percent of marathon runners and other hard-driven, competitive athletes (including cyclists, gymnasts, figure skaters, body builders and dancers, and to a lesser extent, swimmers) have been found to experience irregular, scanty and infrequent periods, mostly without ovulation, or varying intervals of amenorrhea.

Ballet dancers, swimmers, runners and other athlete/performers who start exercising or competing vigorously before they have begun to menstruate often experience a delay in menarche. In a recent study, for example, Dr. Rose E. Frisch of Harvard University and colleagues from other institutions surveyed a group of college-age swimmers and runners. Those who had begun their careers before menstruating experienced their first period at about 15—almost three years later than the national average age for menarche (now 12.3). Those whose training started after first menstruation had entered menarche more or less on schedule. Each year of intensive conditioning before a first period can delay the onset of menarche by five months, the study concluded.

A number of theories have been advanced to explain how and why exercise may markedly tip the menstrual scales. One third of the estrogen circulating in a woman's bloodstream is synthesized by her fatty tissues. Thus, the reduction in body fat that results from any spartan athletic regimen could diminish a woman's estrogen level to a critical point below which ovulation and menstruation will either not occur or only sporadically. Scientists have noted that this reaction to lowered body weight may also be nature's built-in safety valve: ensuring against pregnancy when a woman lacks adequate fat reserves to nourish a developing fetus. Yet, lowered fat ratios cannot account for every case: Many lean women whose fat totals less than 17 percent of their body weight still continue to menstruate. And victims of anorexia nervosa may stop having periods even *before* they have lost a substantial amount of weight.

The mental and emotional stress associated with the rigors of endurance training and the pressures of competition may upset the hormone equilibrium as well. Dr. Mona Shangold, assistant professor of obstetrics and gynecology at the Cornell University Medical Center in New York City observes that women who are physically active every day who do *not* compete are probably less subject to menstrual irregularity than their competitive counterparts, even those involved in considerably less strenuous sports.

In most cases, exercise-related menstrual abnormalities are a strictly temporary condition. Menstruation returns to normal when the strenuous training stops or an athlete approaches her ideal weight. Admittedly, some doctors are still not certain about the long-range effects on young girls whose first periods are significantly delayed by early sports commitment—the lean, record-breaking 12-year-olds who are logging up to 60 to 90 miles a week on the running track. For one thing, postponement of menarche may prolong an adolescent's growth period well into her mid to late teens. (Bones generally stop growing within two years after a girl starts menstruating and releasing reproductive hormones.) This may mean she will wind up far taller than normal, which could affect her self-image, possibly even her relationships with peers or the opposite sex. Another possible result of *excessive* activity is premature bone thinning due to the reduced output of estrogen.

But consider the positive side of the coin: A budding athlete whose menarche is later than average will be at an advantage in almost any sport since height is definitely an athletic asset. Also, in moderation, and along with a proper diet, exercise actually slows down the age-related loss of bone mass which could eventually lead to osteoporosis (see Chapter 5.) Some doctors believe that the advantages of delayed menarche and sports-induced amenorrhea are definitely greater than any drawbacks. In fact, a few experts question whether it is not outright beneficial for the first period to be delayed deliberately, as long as possible! For more on this controversial viewpoint, see p. 60.

THE GOOD NEWS

Very often, women athletes who show up at their gynecologists' offices with menstrual irregularities are told to stop or cut down on their exercise. But the evidence may be purely circumstantial: Disrupted cycles are not necessarily activity-related and doctors should conduct a thorough physical exam to rule out any other possibility. Athletes are not immune to organic disorders such as ovarian failure or pituitary tumors and deserve the same medical consideration as non-athletes. The checkup should include a complete history and measurement of the body's estrogen level. The latter can be done by a number of methods, including an examination of the cervical mucus. When stimulated by estrogen, it becomes clear, colorless, watery, thick and stretchable (a texture called "spinnbarkeit"). A doctor may also measure a patient's BBT (basal body temperature) to determine whether or not she is ovulating.

But another recent look at the menstrual cycles of women athletes has turned up some surprisingly positive news. Dr. Shangold's study of 394 women who ran the New York City marathon showed that 93 percent of those who menstruated regularly before they started running experienced no change after they became marathon competitors. Dr.

Shangold also found that more of the women entrants had monthly irregularities *before* they took up running compared to women in the general population. Maybe the kind of person attracted to this event has a certain degree of drive or other "stress-related factors" that could throw off her menstrual cycle, Dr. Shangold proposes.

Even more interesting was the finding that distance running actually *regulated* cycles in some cases: For 26 percent of the women who were irregular before they began competing, menstrual patterns became normal after training. And 17 percent of those with amenorrhea reported that menstruation resumed once they started exercising! So, according to this report, more women athletes went from being irregular to regular than the other way around. And many could trace their troubled periods to a time *before* they were physically active. While one study alone is not considered conclusive and other surveys have yielded different results, the outcome suggests that the effects of exercise on menstruation may often be therapeutic and that other factors could account for the apparent link between erratic cycles and active women.

Keep in mind that woman have won Olympic Gold medals at all phases of the menstrual cycle. Some athletes report feeling and performing worse during their periods, others claim they do better, and over half have noticed no change at all.

To help keep any exercise-related malfunctions to a minimum, some researchers advise maintaining your cholesterol and protein calorie level at the maximum acceptable amount (cholesterol is one key ingredient from which estrogen is made), keeping weight stable while working out and even possibly curbing your speed at a given sport without reducing your distance.

SHOULD MENARCHE BE DELAYED ON PURPOSE?

Is delayed menarche or temporary amenorrhea in women athletes necessarily undesirable; a "deficiency" which should be corrected at the earliest possible opportunity? Is it a sign of some major disturbance in the reproductive system? According to Robert A. Wild, M.D., director of reproductive endocrinology and fertility service, department of obsetrics and gynecology at the University of Tennessee College of Medicine in Knoxville, the question is certainly open to debate. As he notes in a recent issue of *Medical Aspects of Human Sexuality*, "The reproductive functioning of lean, physically active young women may be more 'normal' than that of their well-nourished, sedentary peers. Indeed, the amenorrhea induced by exercise combined with leanness may be a health *benefit*. Several studies suggested that later menarche and amenorrhea due to excessive leanness may be associated in later life with a lowered risk of breast cancer and possibly also cancer of the endometrium." This stands to reason, as both diseases can arise under the stimulus of too much estrogen, especially when progesterone is relatively deficient. A shutdown of the reproductive system for several years may give these organs a "rest," meaning that a woman is that much less exposed to the continual onslaught of female hormones.

A similar argument can be applied to nutrition and first menstruation. Just as with exercise's effects on the cycle, the assumption that a late menarche is somehow less desirable than an early one has gone unchallenged. Thus, books on menstruation invariably report that the age at the first period has been steadily decreasing due to *improved nutrition* and better living habits. But this earlier menarche may well be the result of certain nutritional *excesses*, such as too much fat or protein and possibly inadequate dietary fiber, any or all of which may stimulate hormone production too early and accelerate the menstrual clock. We may be living and eating more affluently and abundantly today, but that doesn't necessarily mean we are markedly healthier or that we haven't introduced a host of new problems or disorders as a result. For more on this possibility, see the chapter on diet and menstruation.

Caution: Women with chronic, untreated menstrual irregularities due to polycystic ovaries or other anovulatory states may be at a higher than normal risk of breast or endometrial cancer after menopause, reports Dr. Carolyn B. Coulam, director of the Reproductive Endocrinology and Infertility Clinic at the Mayo Clinic in Rochester, Minnesota. Why: Their bodies may be secreting estrogen, but not enough progesterone. Long periods of estrogen production stimulating both breast and endometrial tissue without the counterbalancing effects of progesterone could lead to the development of malignant growths.

This concern apparently does *not* apply to women whose hormone balance has been affected by diet or rigorous athletic training.

Chapter 4

PMS UPDATE:
HAVE YOU COME A LONG WAY, BABY?

"About two years ago, after my son Timothy was born I became very tense and depressed. I also started having angry outbursts at home or on the job for no apparent reason. At the very least I'd snap at my husband and kids, ready to pick a fight over anything, and the most trivial mishaps would reduce me to tears. Other times, I'd be so tired that I would feel like sleeping all day. Nothing seemed to matter except this terrible fatigue . . . Then a week or so later my period would start and my spirits would suddenly lift—dramatically. It was not until then that I'd realize my menstrual cycle was at the bottom of all this."

"It happens without warning! What starts as a beautiful day turns into a real teeth-gritting affair. I feel edgy, irritable and not at all amused! I seem to withdraw into myself and can go on for days without calling friends. I have a heavy, achy sensation in my back and legs, and my rings get tight around my fingers. If I skip a meal I become sweaty and light-headed. No one seems to understand why any of this occurs. Several doctors have suggested tranquilizers but I don't want any medication. Sometimes I feel like I'm out of control . . ."

Many women may suffer similar—and equally baffling—clusters of symptoms some time during each menstrual cycle. Once written off as primarily psychosomatic and rarely or inappropriately treated, their malaise has recently been granted official title and recognition as PMS or "premenstrual syndrome." In fact, some European countries, including Great Britain and France, even permit its consideration in the courts as the basis of "diminished responsibility" for criminal acts.

Unfortunately, however, all this attention has done very little to clear up the confusion—or controversy. Despite the massive media coverage, PMS remains as elusive and poorly understood as ever. No one yet knows precisely how many women suffer from PMS or what causes it or any one surefire way of overcoming the problem. For every study that demonstrates that low levels of progesterone are a primary or contributing factor, there is a report suggesting just the opposite, or showing the influence of some other underlying mechanism. The evidence remains conflicting and inconclusive.

In this chapter, we will try to bring you up to date on everything that has been reported about PMS so far—but we caution you that much of the material is speculative and awaits solid proof or further investigation.

Even if still tentative, however, discussion of PMS can only help speed the process of finding out more about it. We applaud the efforts made already to legitimize the existence of this complaint. We would hope, in fact, that greater awareness among women about premenstrual symptoms will encourage prospective, double-blind studies in the near future that help determine the number of those affected, and how and why they are susceptible, along with the best way to evaluate and treat their condition. If the already established PMS clinics are truly interested in the advancement of medical knowledge, then they should promote such research as well.

While we will describe a number of possible causes and "cures" for PMS in the pages that follow, we would not feel comfortable dogmatically recommending one therapy over another because we simply don't know enough yet.

64

We suggest you discuss any cycle-related symptoms with your doctor and stay well-informed about the latest developments regarding PMS.

Anywhere from one to 14 days before the onset of a period, a still undetermined number of women experience real discomfort in the form of mood and behavioral upsets such as lethargy, depression and extreme irritability and/or strictly physical complaints—among them, headache, bloating, breast tenderness, acne, heart palpitations and unusual hunger pangs. One husband remarks that he knows his (otherwise budget-conscious) wife is nearing her period when she starts "running up whopping bills" at the local bakery! Some studies have estimated that about five percent of women are gripped by severe or debilitating premenstrual problems.

In a recent article in *The Journal of the American Medical Association* (JAMA), Dr. Richard E. Shader, professor and chairman of the department of psychiatry at Tufts University School of Medicine, reports that "premenstrual syndrome may be the newest women's health issue in the United States. Some severely affected women are now going public with their stories and are demanding treatment . . . The *small minority* whose lives are *seriously* disrupted (emphasis ours) reputedly may experience exacerbations of chronic medical illnesses, abuse their children or commit violent crimes. Some are said to be suicidal."

PMS is most likely to arise during times of hormonal upheaval—at puberty or after pregnancy, for example, and may become progressively worse with age. The patterns and timing of the syndrome vary from woman to woman. Thus, some experience a dramatic onrush of symptoms at ovulation, followed by a completely trouble-free interval, then a return to even more serious distress about a week before menstruation. Others feel their worst about four or five days before the flow. For a few, unfortunately, misery erupts with full force at ovulation and does not subside until the first several days of the period roughly two weeks later.

This mercurial disorder does not necessarily occur at the

same time each month nor with the same degree of severity. Diet, stress, lifestyle and other influences determine the intensity of symptoms in women who are susceptible. Though the discomfort may taper off gradually, it often ends quite abruptly and, in fact, the relief has been described by such phrases as "a cloud lifts" and "in an instant I know I'm going to be fine."

PMS: WHAT TO LOOK FOR

Before examining the causes of PMS and the ways it can be prevented, you should be aware of its wide-ranging possible symptoms which are known to occur collectively and—primarily for convenience and easy reference—may be divided into several categories: These are based on what are believed to be the underlying physiological conditions that give rise to each complaint, though no one knows for sure.

Water Retention

Abdominal bloating (The motility of intestines is altered, leading to swelling, constipation, heaviness)
Breast tenderness
Leg and ankle swelling
Water weight gain
Backache, congestive low back pain, "draggy" feeling in thighs and back
Joint pain
Migraines
Dizziness or vertigo
Acute sensitivity to light and noise
Sinusitis
Glaucoma-like symptoms and other visual disturbances resulting from intraocular edema (swelling within eye region)

Sodium/Potassium Imbalance

Tension

Depression
Irritability
Lethargy
Fatigue, generally weak or "washed out" feeling
Arrhythmia (heart palpitations, occasional irregular beats)
Muscle weakness (leading to possible clumsiness and poor coordination. Some women are believed to be slightly more accident-prone or less muscularly efficient during their premenstrual phase as a result.)

Metabolic Disturbances

Headaches
Lightheadedness or fainting
Irritability
Hunger pangs, cravings for sweets or salty foods, possible binging
Nausea
Exhaustion, sleepiness
Aggressive behavior
Tearful outbursts
Mood swings
Insomnia
Lethargy
Difficulty concentrating
Greater susceptibility to alcohol
Panic attacks (could mimic agoraphobia)
Suicidal feelings

Lowered Resistance to Infection

Upper respiratory infections, greater likelihood of colds, sore throats, etc.
Rhinitis
Skin eruptions or rashes
Acne flareups
Conjunctivitis
Boils
Herpes recurrences
Asthma attacks
Allergic reactions

Bleeding gums, more bruising
Bladder irritations

Prostaglandin Excess or Deficiency

Changes in urination (more frequent or less)
Constipation
Diarrhea
Nausea, vomiting
Digestive upsets
Abdominal cramps
Breast tenderness
Low back pain
Weight gain
Fluid retention
Visual disturbances

In the past, a woman who complained to her doctor of persistent headaches or lethargy or crying spells was often treated with anti-depressants and other medications. Rarely was any connection made between her condition and the timing of her menstrual cycle—the question, "When are you expecting your period?" was simply never asked.

"Tranquilizers made me feel *worse*," one woman recalls. "I was completely 'strung out.' My doctor also gave me a diuretic to relieve the bloating but I felt so fatigued as a result that I was unable to function normally. Next, he put me on birth control pills and the symptoms returned with a vengeance—more intense than ever. I thought I was going crazy!"

These prescriptions didn't work—and rather created new problems—because they were designed to treat symptoms only, instead of considering them connected to any underlying cause. Now that we are more aware that complaints of depression, tearfulness or erratic mood swings may sometimes be related to a troubled monthly cycle, the above scenario should be far less likely. Medical history-taking will include questions to help determine whether or not a woman's problem is premenstrual.

WHAT CAUSES PMS?

Among the many interesting theories, one frequently cited is that PMS may result from a relative deficiency of progesterone compared with estrogen—either excess estrogen production by the ovaries or else too little progesterone secreted by the corpus luteum. (See Chapter 1.) The timing of estrogen/progesterone release may also be off, disrupting the delicate hormone balance that regulates the monthly cycle.

It has been reported that a relative shortage of progesterone may affect the body's capacity to metabolize carbohydrates (sugars and starches) which could account for some particularly stressful symptoms. Low progesterone is also considered partly responsible for excess fluid retention.

A study at St. Thomas Hospital in London conducted by Professor Lawrence Taylor and Dr. Michael Brush found that the progesterone level in 40 percent of the women who suffered from PMS was not as high as it should have been at a critical point in their cycle—when progesterone is normally at its peak to stimulate further development of the uterine lining.[1] The researchers also found that nearly the same percentage of women—some of whom *did* show adequate progesterone—had elevated blood levels of *estrogen*, which upset the ratio between the two hormones. When progesterone was lower than normal, the surplus of estrogen probably made the hormonal discrepancy even worse.

Several other factors contribute to the belief that lopsided hormones are at least one primary cause of PMS, as Judy Lever and Dr. Michael Brush explain in their book, *Premenstrual Tension*. For example, the syndrome "only occurs on those days of the cycle when progesterone *should* be present, and at a relatively high level. After menstruation, when progesterone drops off naturally anyway, the symp-

---

[1]*Premenstrual Tension* by Judy Lever with Dr. Michael G. Brush, McGraw-Hill Book Co., New York, 1981, pp. 39–40.

toms *never* occur." And there is a notable absence of complaints during pregnancy, when high levels of progesterone are produced by the placenta to nourish the growing embryo.

Vitamin B6 or pyridoxine is involved in the proper release of estrogen and progesterone and below-average levels of the vitamin are reportedly another characteristic of some women with premenstrual syndrome. Inadequate pyridoxine is believed to disrupt the hypothalamus/pituitary connection which can lead to a number of brain-chemical imbalances such as low levels of serotonin (a possible cause of depression) and of dopamine. Too little dopamine can result in an excess of *prolactin*, a hormone that can adversely affect the ovaries and breasts, and maybe the body's fluid balance as well.[2] Since the hypothalamus itself controls weight, appetite, moods, fluid levels and other metabolic states, anything that impairs its proper functioning could trigger troubling premenstrual symptoms.

The omnipresent prostaglandins are also thought to play a rather paradoxical role in the origins of PMS. Some recent evidence suggests that both a deficiency of a certain beneficial prostaglandin and an oversupply of the more detrimental kind may account for a number of common complaints.

A shortage of an essential fatty acid, gamma-linolenic acid, may lower the supply of prostaglandin E (PGE1), a hormone-like chemical which monitors the health of almost every cell in the body. A relative absence of PGE1 may precipitate some of the symptoms associated with PMS including breast tenderness, fluid retention, weight gain, low back pain and visual disturbances. Linolenic acid cannot be manufactured by the body so an adequate amount must be provided by the diet. Besides human milk, the richest available natural source is the oil extracted from the evening primrose flower (Efamol). By offering a daily regimen of Efamol (along with careful attention to diet and other important nutrients), Drs. Donald Lombard and

[2]*Premenstrual Tension*, p. 42.

Ann Nazzarro, who run Mill River Clinical Associates in Northampton, Massachusetts, have claimed remarkable success in treating sufferers with PMS. (Bear in mind that Efamol is a rather expensive treatment.)

The hormone prolactin produces changes in mood and fluid metabolism similar to those which arise in PMS. In fact, some women with elevated premenstrual prolactin levels find symptomatic relief with a powerful prescription drug called bromocriptine (Parlodel) which suppresses prolactin release. Most women with PMS have *normal* levels of prolactin. But some researchers have found that when PGE1 is relatively low, body tissues are unusually sensitive to even normal amounts of prolactin—which may have the same effect as an excess of the troublesome hormone.

The "good" prostaglandin theory may also help explain why two other nutritional therapies, vitamin B6 and magnesium, have been reported partially effective in controlling PMS. Both nutrients help the body convert its essential fatty acids to PGE1, thereby boosting its supply of this crucial element.

Some physicians believe that a surplus of undesirable prostaglandins could be responsible for premenstrual distress as well. The shifting ratios of estrogen, progesterone and prolactin during the latter part of the cycle may raise the number of these wrong-headed prostaglandins to uncomfortable levels. The possible results include pain, nausea, digestive and abdominal discomfort, tenderness, headaches and cramping, as well as changes in brain chemistry which could affect monthly moods.

As reported in the chapter on dysmenorrhea (menstrual cramps), the total prostaglandin level *does* increase during the premenstrual phase, and drops off sharply with the onset of flow—so this may well be a leading instigator in PMS. The presence of prolactin itself steps up the output of "bad" prostaglandins, and a relative shortage of progesterone may also keep the PG level unnaturally high.

ALL IN YOUR HEAD?

The so-called emotional disturbances that have been attributed to PMS, including irritability, temper outbursts, nervous tension, depression and even panic attacks may stem from possible premenstrual instability in the blood sugar level or a temporary hypoglycemia-like condition in some women. This may be brought on by the estrogen/progesterone imbalance. (Why the same kind of bodily response may give rise to lethargy and sullenness in one woman and hyperactive or aggressive behavior in another is still not yet fully understood, though both reactions are plausible effects of a sudden, abnormal or unusually sustained decline in the blood sugar level.)

Carbohydrates, proteins and fats are digested or converted into "sugar" or glucose, our natural source of energy. After a meal, the level of this body fuel rises and then slowly drops back down, which sends hunger signals to the brain, once again prompting us to eat. If you are not premenstrual and you go on for extended periods without eating, your body will compensate for the lowered blood sugar level by secreting *adrenalin*, which causes the liver to release glucose directly into the bloodstream. Adrenalin, the notorious "fight or flight" hormone which the body normally summons during a sudden emergency, danger or stressful event, results in an accelerated heart rate, heightened blood pressure, excitability, nervous tension and anxiety. This hormone-triggered response may be experienced as irritability, difficulty in breathing, palpitations, insomnia, dizziness, faintness, panic and easy distractibility. Even migraine headaches and epileptic seizures have been linked to the adrenalin response.

In their premenstrual phase, some women may experience biochemical changes which decrease the amount that their blood sugar level has to fall *before* adrenalin is released and with it, the unsettling symptoms. Thus, hormonal shifts during this interval may make some of us more sensitive to *smaller* drops in blood sugar.[3] In many premenstrual women, the response to such "lowered glucose tolerance" is a craving for sweets not long after a meal. These insatiable pangs can weaken the resolve of even the most dedicated weight-watcher. So dieting calls for extra vigilance in this case, and the irony is that *not* eating at the right time may cause the whole problem in the first place!

To stabilize the body's metabolism pre-menstrually I recommend eating about six small meals throughout the day instead of three normal-sized ones. *Never* fast or skip meals and dine as slowly and leisurely as possible. This will help fuel your body with a more constant supply of food which it can convert to glucose at a steady rate.

The best choices are meals rich in protein and complex carbohydrates which take longer to be metabolized than simple, refined starches and sugars and can therefore deliver a more long-term dose of energy. In addition, these items are more plentiful in vitamins, minerals and fiber which have been processed out of other foods.

Probably the worst foods for premenstrual symptoms are highly refined sugars and flours (white bread and rolls, pastries, cookies, white rice, sweetened soft drinks, ice cream, candies and the like.) Since such foods require little or no breakdown, they very quickly enter the bloodstream and just as rapidly are consumed, possibly giving way to an abrupt decline in glucose to the hunger level. Also, steer clear of substances such as caffeine and alcohol which may alter the free sugars circulating in the blood and cause the glucose to dip faster than normal.

[3]Information provided by doctors at the *PMS Medical Group* in New York City (a Center for the treatment of premenstrual syndrome. For further details, contact PMS Medical Group, Lincoln Towers, Suite 1G, 140 West End Avenue, New York, NY 10023.

THAT WATER-LOGGED FEELING

As mentioned above, water retention resulting from an upset in the sodium/potassium equilibrium, an imbalance between estrogen and progesterone, a prostaglandin deficiency or some other factor, underlies yet another familiar cluster of premenstrual conditions: most commonly, weight gain, swelling and heaviness in legs, ankles, feet, abdomen and breasts, along with joint and back pain and certain headaches. Tissues of the face (especially near the eyes and ears), fingers or gums may be painful and tender because accumulated fluids have led to stretching.

High estrogen relative to progesterone binds sodium in the body which has a fluid-retaining effect. When delicate brain membranes fill up with this excess water, the result is pain and possible dizziness, a so-called "estrogen headache."

Another symptom related to fluid buildup is a prickly, tingling sensation in the hands and fingers arising from the constriction of nerves by water-logged tissues in the wrist (known as the carpal tunnel syndrome). Watching the bathroom scale register a monthly increase of as much as four to 12 pounds (of excess water) may itself generate depression and irritability, especially in women who are trying to lose weight and are repeatedly frustrated in their attempt during premenstrual days. (See Chapter 8 on diet and the menstrual cycle.)

The widespread practice of prescribing diuretics to counteract water weight will actually aggrevate rather than relieve one of the recognized disturbances of the premenstrual period. While holding back water and sodium, the body excretes potassium in the urine. Diuretics by their nature itensify this potassium loss which may leave the body critically depleted of this necessary chemical. Shortage of potassium is known to cause feelings of fatigue and muscle weakness, familiar premenstrual complaints.

Even the mildest prescription of diuretics, sparingly used, could have this undesirable effect. One, called Dyrenium (generic name, triamterene) is so far the best choice because it does not result in significant potassium loss. If you must resort to diuretics, supplement your diet with bananas and oranges, two natural sources of potassium. Avoid increasing your coffee intake and try gradually switching to decaffeinated brands since caffeine is itself a strong diuretic. It also heightens the nervous tension associated with PMS. Note: Natural dietary diuretics include cranberry juice or the freshly extracted juices of such vegetables as celery, cucumber, asparagus and watercress.

TRANQUILIZERS: THE WRONG WAY

Knowing the causes of PMS will enable you to understand just why certain medications such as tranquilizers, diuretics and birth control pills don't work and in fact could aggravate your symptoms.

For example, the chief drawback of such tranquilizers as Valium and Librium—especially when given in excessive amounts or for too long a period of time—is that they may increase the lethargy, drowsiness, weakness and nervous system depression already suffered by many victims of PMS, explains Dr. Joseph Martoranno, a psychopharmacologist affiliated with the PMS Medical Group in New York City. Tranquilizers also increase the level of prolactin, the pituitary hormone that depresses progesterone, and so may intensify existing premenstrual symptoms.

The goal in treating patients with any menstrual complaint is to help them function and perform at their best, whether at home or on the job—which makes sedation a questionable, last-resort therapy. The experience of many physicians indicates that a well-planned dietary regimen combined with certain nutritional supplements and possibly other presumed PMS relievers like antiprostaglandins, natural progesterone and gamma linolenic acid can work successfully, reducing or eliminating the need for tranquilizers altogether.

The fluctuations of mood that characterize some cases of

PMS have sometimes been diagnosed as manic-depressive illness, which has led to treatment with lithium. While this drug can minimize mood swings, depression or temperamental outbursts by helping to restore the body to its normal fluid balance, it loses its effectiveness with prolonged use and carries the risk of serious side effects. Thus, as with other antidepressants and tranquilizers, lithium should *never* be prescribed routinely for PMS unless there are other psychiatric indications for its use.

Some women have been misdiagnosed with such labels as alcoholic, agoraphobic and manic-depressive and then subsequently treated with powerful, mind-altering drugs which have worsened their PMS symptoms, Dr. Martoranno points out. As a result, a physician may have switched drugs or resorted to even more potent formulas in the search for lasting relief. Meanwhile, he or she may not have asked that all-important question about the possible relationship of the patient's disorders to the phase of her menstrual cycle.

If antidepressants are prescribed, they generally take three weeks to work. Thus, if a woman started taking them, say, a week before her period, by the time they took effect, she might be nearing her premenstrual time when her complaints would again be at their peak. This apparent flareup of symptoms could convince her doctor to increase the drug dosage or else to try another antidepressant. And the probable side effects of such therapy would only make the premenstrual problem *worse*.

Why was PMS an invisible syndrome for so long? The multiplicity of reported ills were hard to connect with any one physiological phenomenon (or even with several for that matter), until physicians found out more about the impact of crucial hormone shifts and other factors on the female body and its delicate cycles. Often, too, patients initially complaining of fatigue, migraines and "low blood sugar" would make it to the doctor's office only when they were feeling considerably better (probably after they started menstruating)—once the miserable, stay-at-home symptoms were gone! If they were given a blood sugar tolerance test at this point, results would be negative, of course—possibly leading a doctor to conclude that these and other complaints were nonexistent or largely imagined.

On the other hand, a premenstrual sufferer may have visited her physician complaining of intermittent panic attacks or palpitations. If not alert to the possibility of PMS, he might reasonably assume she was stricken with anxiety or agoraphobia and prescribe a beta blocker called propranolol (Inderal) to relieve the symptoms. However, while the attacks would inevitably subside with the onset of menstruation, their disappearance would be wrongly credited to the Inderal rather than to the natural "upswing" in the menstrual cycle! No one, not even the patient herself, would necessarily make any connection between the advent of the flow and the relief of the symptoms.

Both the mechanics of the menstrual cycle and the possibility of misdiagnosis may explain in part why 10 women to every man have experienced panic attacks associated with and frequently identified as agoraphobia, argues Dr. Martoranno.

Birth control pills can actually worsen PMS in some women whose symptoms result from a relative deficiency of progesterone, according to Katharina Dalton of England, who is credited with the pioneering work on PMS and claims to have successfully treated it for the past 30 years. The reason: Oral contraceptives contain *synthetic* progesterone which completely suppresses the natural progesterone in the body, as well as providing synthetic estrogen while raising the level of estrogen. Thus, women with untreated PMS often add yet another problem to their list—inability to tolerate the Pill.

Dr. Dalton has reported excellent results by administering natural progesterone, a substance grown from yams which is similar to what the body makes on its own. It is given either by injection or suppository. (The natural hormone is broken down quickly by digestive enzymes and so is ineffective when taken orally.)

There are no known risks to such treatment so far,* and there are reports of 50 to 70 percent of women with initially severe symptoms who claim significant relief within the first month. However, unless your problems are extreme and debilitating, you can probably manage PMS effectively without resorting to expensive hormone therapy. In a majority of cases, the right nutritional routine can correct the physiological imbalances—whether too little progesterone, a shortage or surplus of prostaglandins, vitamin or mineral deficiencies or some combination of these—that are causing your discomfort. Aerobic and relaxation exercises along with anti-stress techniques will further help keep PMS under control. For those women who still require progesterone for complete relief, a rectal solution is easier to administer than a suppository and can be just as effective at a lower dose.

OVERCOMING PMS: THE BEST SOLUTIONS

Progesterone, responsible for further developing the uterine lining already prepared by estrogen, is broken down into two by-products (aldosterone and deoxycortisone) which have strong sodium and water-retaining effects on the kidneys. A woman experiencing the stress of severe PMS may release more aldosterone than normal along with an even more powerful water-retaining hormone called anti-diuretic hormone. As you have seen, the all-too-familiar physiological effects include engorged and tender breasts, abdominal swelling, weight gain, less frequent urination and/or swollen ankles, feet and hands. Fluids may also collect in areas where the tissues cannot stretch to accommodate them, resulting in an unnatural pressure buildup in the skull and eye area, inner ear, spinal discs or nerves of

---

*One possible inconvenience is occasional breakthrough bleeding.

the wrists. The consequences could be migraines, acute eyeball pain, dizziness, backache and numbness in the fingers, among other problems.

You may note a substantial easing of such symptoms simply by cutting down on the sodium in your diet. You can do this by eliminating canned, frozen, pickled, preserved and prepackaged foods, and reading labels carefully for sodium content. Highly salted foods include artichokes, sauerkraut, spinach, chard, kale, beets, herring, lobster, shellfish, scallops, bacon, frankfurters, sausages, cold cuts, organ meats, nuts, pretzels, popcorn, some breakfast cereals and cakes. Also watch out for instant hot chocolate, MSG, bouillon cubes, catsup, mustard, relishes, olives, pickles, soy and Worchestershire sauces, frozen pizza and pudding mixes. Use fresh herbs and spices for flavor instead of salt. Steam vegetables to preserve their natural taste and nutritional content, and season them with freshly squeezed lemon juice or tarragon vinegar.

Remember, the average American's salt intake is already 10 to 20 times what is required for optimum health—so family members will certainly benefit from any salt-restricting regimen. (It should serve as a guideline for lifelong eating.) Happily, there is an abundance of low-sodium foods from which to choose and around which to plan your menus. These include fresh fruits, many cereals, cabbage, broccoli, corn, peppers, potatoes, beans, pastas, lean lamb, chicken, fish packed in water and freshly made sauces or condiments.

Along with sodium vigilance, follow the dietary guidelines already suggested, calling for frequent small meals with emphasis on protein and complex carbohydrates to ensure a fairly steady release of blood sugar throughout the day. Good quality protein choices are low-fat dairy products, seafood, poultry, lean meats, grains and legumes. Complex carbohydrates are the whole-grain breads, cereals and pastas, brown rice, starchy fresh vegetables and fruits.

Premenstrual headaches are sometimes thought to be the result of metabolic disturbances such as blood sugar fluctuations or sensitivities to certain foods. When the blood sugar is relatively low, the body often compensates for the deficiency by sending a greater volume of blood to the brain. The result of this higher pressure and "stretching" of blood vessels could be throbbing head pain. Similarly, the sensitive body may overreact to certain foods by producing digestive residues called amines which dilate capillaries and increase both circulation and pressure within tissues of the brain. Such amines are naturally found in aged cheeses (cheddar, Parmesan, processed cheese foods), red wine, sherry, port, champagne, herring and chocolate. Citrus fruits, gluten flour, onions, pork, ripe bananas and shellfish may also trigger amine-type reactions during the premenstrual phase.

Caffeine is well-known for aggravating certain symptoms of PMS because of several undesirable side effects. For one thing, it boosts the body's level of troublemaking prostaglandins; these may be at least partly responsible for breast tenderness, abdominal discomfort, headaches, cramping, backaches and joint pain. A vigorous diuretic, caffeine could reduce the body's supply of essential nutrients such as potassium, magnesium and water-soluble vitamins, which may be at lower-than-normal levels in victims of PMS, who experience fatigue, depression and irritability as a result. Caffeine may also stimulate adrenalin release and destabilize blood sugar levels, thereby intensifying nervous tension, tremors, insomnia, palpitations, concentration difficulties, fatigue or irritability.

Don't cut out caffeine cold-turkey style, however, since withdrawal symptoms include throbbing headaches and other problems which will only reinforce or mimic premenstrual distress. To taper off gradually, begin by reducing your coffee, tea and cola drinking by one cup a day. Keep in mind that coarser grinds of coffee have a lower caffeine content than finer blends, and the amount also varies according to the method of preparation, with dripolated topping the list, followed by percolated, regular instant and decaffeinated instant. Herbal teas and Postum are good substitutes. If coffee drinking has become a mindless ritual, try keeping track of where, when and with whom you indulge and what mood you're in at the time to help you avoid certain habit-forming situations.

VITAMIN AND
MINERAL SUPPLEMENTS

Two vitamins that may relieve PMS ills are B6 and A. A key brain-cell nutrient, B6 plays a role in the proper assimilation or breakdown of amino acids (the components of proteins) and is necessary in adequate amounts for the production of estrogen and progesterone. As already noted, a shortage of B6 is believed to *decrease* the prolactin-inhibiting brain chemical dopamine, and likewise the mood-elevating serotonin with possibly unfortunate results.

Since the B vitamins are water-soluble, they are not stored in the body and any excess will be excreted in the urine. Some physicians recommend taking the vitamin at least three days before expected symptoms and continuing until three days into the menstrual period—starting typically with 50 mgs. a day and increasing this up to 200 mgs. until you notice results. (At higher dosages, you may risk some mild gastric acidity, the only worrisome possible side effect.) Pyridoxine should be taken in its B-complex form, not alone, because in high doses it tends to deplete the other B vitamins in the body.

Natural food sources of B6 include whole-grain breads and cereals, cabbage and other fresh vegetables, rice, Brewer's yeast, milk and eggs. Sleeping pills, caffeine, alcohol, sulfa drugs and estrogen (the Pill) are all B6 consumers and therefore dependence on any of these will raise your body's requirements for the vitamin.

Vitamin A has a mild diuretic effect and so may partly relieve swelling of the breasts and lower abdomen. It is also an immune system strengthener which may help ward off stress and fatigue. Vitamin C, too, may help sustain

81

resistance to upper respiratory ailments and has been shown to limit both the severity and duration of cold symptoms. Since heightened susceptibility to infection is among the array of maladies associated with PMS, supplementing your diet with extra C (up to 500 to 1,000 mgs. daily) is also a good idea.

The richest food sources of vitamin A include the golden-fleshed vegetables and fruits, particularly squash, yams, carrots, peaches, nectarines and apricots, along with dairy products, egg yolks and liver.

Many American women are considered to have chronically low levels of the minerals calcium, magnesium and potassium. Stress and poor dietary habits are primarily to blame. When sustained and excessive, stress can release an abnormal amount of lactic acid into the bloodstream which binds calcium in the blood and makes it unavailable to the nervous system where it is needed most, along with muscle and bone cells. A calcium shortage can show up as weakness and depression or excitability and anxiety.

Stress also results in the manufacture of certain hormones which accelerate magnesium loss via urine and hamper our digestive system's capacity to absorb magnesium and other minerals from the foods we eat, In one nutritional study, women with PMS showed a lower magnesium level between body cells than women who were symptom-free. Potassium, too, is particularly essential to the control of PMS as levels of this mineral decline when sodium and water are retained premenstrually.

Food sources of calcium are the dairy products: skim milk, low-fat yogurt, pot, farmer, feta cheese and low-sodium cheeses (advisable for those with bloating problems). Other excellent sources are dark green and yellow vegetables such as broccoli, asparagus, squash and zucchini. (Vegetables should be raw or minimally cooked, with little water, preferably steamed or stir-fried.) Magnesium is found in whole-grain breads and cereals, nuts, nut butters and fresh green vegetables. Potassium is supplied by bananas, oranges, tomatoes, apricots and fresh fruit or vegetable juices.

EXERCISE AND PMS

Probably one of the most effective antidotes to PMS is sustained, vigorous exercise—the kind that gets the pulse rate up and keeps it there. Best examples: swimming, cycling, jogging, rebounding, rope-skipping and aerobic dancing. Over a period of months, aerobic workouts not only condition the cardiovascular system, but also help the body metabolize carbohydrates more efficiently. In addition, exercise releases beta-endorphins, morphine-like chemicals in the body which have a naturally mood-enhancing effect—accounting for the widely reported "runner's high."

Physical activity also decreases fluid and sodium retention, stimulates a sluggish digestive tract and tones abdominal muscles, so it can curb some of the more distressing symptoms of PMS. No one can discount the intangible psychological boost that comes simply from being in top condition, and from the sense of accomplishment and mastery that follow.

As for still other benefits, exercise dissipates body tensions which may erupt as irritability, muscular aches or troubled sleep during premenstrual days. Aerobic activity combined with stretching routines will help muscles stay loose and relaxed, paving the way for more restful sleep and less susceptibility to cramping pain.

For maximum benefit, you should exercise consistently, at least 20 to 30 minutes every other day, and make sure your pulse rate rises to 75 to 80 percent of your aerobic "training" level—roughly calculated by subtracting your age from 220. Thus, a 30-year-old woman should try to get her heart rate to 80 percent of 190 or about 152 beats per minute during the time she is working out.

If you have been sedentary a long time or are strictly a "weekend" athlete, begin slowly and check with your physician first to help determine your most appropriate starting level. Remember that both warm-up and cool-down activities—the proper "before and after" strategies—are crucial to the success and safety of any exercise program.

For those who need another incentive to begin a serious routine of physical activity, keep in mind that after age 35, your body tends to lose one half pound of lean (muscle) tissue while simultaneously gaining a pound of fat every year. Regular exercise can greatly slow down this unwanted replacement.

Along with diet and exercise, simple changes in living habits and some extra self-consideration may be all that's necessary to relieve the not-so-drastic cases of PMS—that means the vast majority! If you feel like resting more, give in to your body's signals. You may experience a general slowdown at this time, so try to eliminate as many outside stressors as possible. Don't overload your schedule with too many high-pressure business sessions or dinner parties—good policy, in fact, any time of the month. Learning to relax can bring about beneficial changes in body chemistry which will help you manage stress more efficiently, with less wear and tear on your system.

Eat 20 minutes before a meeting to keep blood sugar up and both energy and mental powers at their peak. Take naps, relaxation breaks and long leisurely baths to defuse any undue tension.

Fighting off an urge to rest and unwind, or ignoring your physical and emotional symptoms will only make matters worse. Also, let family and friends know what's bothering you so they will understand why you may be unaccountably cranky or out-of-sorts. Unburdening yourself and staying in touch can be a great relief for everybody.

CHARTING YOURSELF

For best results, regardless of how severe your symptoms and what therapy you choose, keep a careful record of your physical and emotional complaints throughout the month as you experience them and the day of the cycle on which they occur. Observe carefully to see if any telltale pattern develops over several cycles.

It will help to take your basal body temperature (BBT) to determine when ovulation has occurred. Progesterone, which is released in noticeable amounts at ovulation, may raise the body's temperature by about a half to one full degree Fahrenheit, so any increase in the thermometer reading should indicate that you have reached your mid-cycle point, after which PMS symptoms may surface. (Take your temperature rectally *before* you get out of bed in the morning and allow about five minutes for the thermometer to register).

You might use a numerical charting system indicating shifting mood levels with figures from 0 to 10, ranging from low to high (your very best days). Self-monitoring can simply help you and your doctor identify your condition, decide which treatment is most appropriate and evaluate the effectiveness of any given regimen.

PMS: ITS IMPLICATIONS

No doubt, PMS may be a convenient catch-all for the hypochondriac, a new, medically validated syndrome on which to pin her present-day ills. Certainly the nebulous and numerous possible complaints defy easy diagnosis. That's why careful record-keeping of the menstrual cycle and corresponding symptoms is important, along with an examination by your gynecologist to determine whether your condition is in fact premenstrual.

Has the woman's movement suffered a setback as a result of the more sensational revelations about PMS? Won't people be able to justify their refusal to grant us equal pay and power on the grounds that we are too biologically fragile and unreliable to be entrusted with certain high-level responsibilities? Is it fair to exonerate some women for criminal acts because they were proven to be suffering from PMS—a disorder so diffuse and wide-ranging that it may account for almost *any* type of behavior?

As for the facts: Two landmark legal decisions in Britain received much of the headline-making publicity about PMS and its link to violent crime. In one case, a scullery maid who had been convicted of stabbing another woman to death was placed on probation because of "mitigating circumstances" attributed to PMS. Another woman ran down her lover with a car, killing him by pinning him against a telephone pole. The original charge of murder was reduced to manslaughter on the grounds of "diminished responsibility" due to PMS. An American woman lawyer was planning to use the PMS argument in a recent child-abuse case, though she withdrew this defense before the trial began.

What is the effect of this new biological rationale for women's behavior, both in and out of court? It can be seen as a victory, in one sense, because what was so persistently regarded as "all in our heads" is now being taken seriously, as a legitimate condition, with a set of specific physiological causes. As a result (just as with dysmenorrhea), effective relief for the symptoms may now be available, obviously an improvement over past neglect.

It's downright comforting to know that some problems, when they *do* occur, have a physical basis; that we are not just suffering from something nameless and uncontrollable. Katherina Dalton's aim was actually to *dispel* the image of women as "uncertain, fickle, moody and changeable" by attributing our long-presumed emotional frailties to the vagaries of basic body chemistry. Women can no longer be dismissed as high-strung or hysterical if they are in the grip of a real disorder.

The new fear that women will be regarded as prisoners of their hormones if truth about PMS leaks out is exaggerated. For one thing, the number of women who commit violent crimes is a very small percentage of the population. Of these, only a handful could even be considered PMS-related, so hormone-triggered criminal acts are extreme cases, indeed. (And at least some women who are inclined to aggressive, self-destructive or bizarre behavior during their premenstrual days may well be unstable to begin with; the hormonal "fuel" might simply cause a latent tendency to erupt full force.) All the media attention, of course, has made this seem more like a female epidemic. Fortunately, the novelty of premenstrual malaise is beginning to wear thin, which should soon put everything in its proper perspective.

If properly and responsibly reported, news about PMS should *not* denigrate women at all. The relative handful of those who are believed to suffer from intense, debilitating symptoms should not be viewed as a source of embarrassment to the women's movement, but rather as deserving of further study and prompt relief. It *is* upsetting when the sufferings of a few are headlined as typical of most women or when they are presumed to be untreatable except with numbing, "knockout" drugs. Just because the majority of us get by with minimal premenstrual discomfort, if any, however, doesn't mean we shouldn't try to recognize and remedy the problem when it does arise. (No one really argues otherwise.)

If biology isn't our destiny, neither should it be overlooked entirely. By ignoring cyclical changes (as if these in themselves could ever be demeaning) we may be ironically siding with those, male or female, who are too squeamish or ill-at-ease to discuss menstruation, menopause or other realities defined by our cycle; who thereby imply that femaleness is somehow not worthy of much analysis or attention. Coverups never work very well, anyway: Instead of trying to silence PMS out of existence, we should see to it that its story is accurately told, not sensationalized, and that we have the means and motivation to find out all the answers.

As for the PMS legal "precedent": This was publicized way out of proportion to its significance. Contrary to some speculation, it is not likely to lead to a rash of similar cases in court since any defense lawyer would have a tricky time proving that his client has the syndrome and committed a crime while under its influence, or had severe enough symptoms to render her behavior beyond control. As the disorder is more readily understood and treated whenever necessary, such cases should become legal rarities anyway. Does PMS make for a fair defense? If it is properly demonstrated and documented, it should be no less fair than is the temporary insanity plea for either sex or the mitigating circumstances due to the intoxicating influence of alcohol or drugs.

Men are far more prone to violent acts and equally susceptible to plain bad moods. As Dr. Dalton has reportedly remarked, "We're better off for our 'raging hormones' than men are for their steady ones." At least a woman can now point to a possible physical reason for some of her unpleasant moods, some of the time. She can even predict her less-than-peak moments and plan her schedule accordingly; a man has no such advantage.

Since the vast majority of premenstrual symptoms can be successfully treated or prevented, publicity about PMS should succeed in calling it to everyone's attention—the women who are profoundly afflicted or even mildly annoyed, along with their physicians and families—so it can be properly identified and ultimately brought under control. In fact, the more said about PMS, the greater the chances that it will eventually disappear.

Chapter 5

MENOPAUSE AND BEYOND

"Several times a day I feel a fiery sensation in my upper throat and face—as if I'm suddenly blushing for no reason. I start perspiring very heavily and even a flimsy, high-necked blouse is downright uncomfortable. Sure enough, a few of my colleagues have noticed that I've looked 'embarrassed' or 'agitated' lately," a 49-year-old editor tells her doctor. "I know this probably means I'm reaching my menopause—but one thing really puzzles me. My periods seem to be coming more frequently lately and they are often heavy and prolonged. I thought just the opposite was supposed to happen!"

"Everyone talks about the 'change of life' but here I am at 55. I'm no longer menstruating, yet otherwise I don't feel very different! I don't remember having a single hot flash or any other symptoms out of the ordinary. Is there something wrong with me or has the whole menopause story been exaggerated?" another woman asks.

No two women experience menopause exactly the same way. As with menstruation itself, the endpoint of a woman's reproductive cycle—the cessation of fertility and monthly flow—is the culmination of a complex chain of biological events beginning several years before the final period.

Aptly labeled the "climacteric," the interval of subtle and gradual changes preceding the menopause results from the slow-but-steady decline of ovarian function. At birth, the ovaries shelter nearly a half million eggs, but the amount dramatically diminishes with age, and only about 400 are ripened and released during a lifetime. By the time a woman reaches her 40s, she may have only about 50 or 60 left, which will be depleted in another several years.

With fewer functioning follicles, the ovaries' output of estrogen and progesterone is reduced as well. Eventually, the hormone levels are simply not high enough to stimulate either ovulation or monthly periods, and the potential for childbearing ends. The effects of this hormone shift range from barely perceptible to nearly incapacitating—with most experiences falling between the two extremes.

Without adequate estrogen, the vagina does not lubricate as quickly when sexually aroused—taking minutes instead of seconds; irritation and infection are more likely as the lining thins out. Headaches, palpitations, hot flashes in the chest, neck and face, sometimes accompanied by drenching sweats and chills; loss of firmness or sensitivity in the breasts, numbness or tingling of the skin and weakening, readily fractured bones (osteoporosis) are among the other possible consequences of estrogen loss. Since this hormone helps shape the female figure and determine the distribution of fat, its withdrawal often triggers weight gain and a change in contour: Fat accumulates around the waist and back, while hips and breasts may lose tissue.

However, a number of women continue to produce and store enough estrogen from their adrenal glands, fatty tissues and the other layer of the ovaries to experience only minimal disturbances, if any. It seems to be the *rate* at which the body stops secreting estrogen that decides the severity of menopause symptoms. If the hormone tapers off gradually and if other sources continue to supply it, the so-called change of life should be virtually trouble-free. The more abrupt the decline, the greater the upheaval. (In fact, premature or "instant" menopause will occur if the ovaries are severely injured in an accident or surgically removed.)

The age at menopause is usually anywhere from 45 to 55, though about eight percent of women reach it before turning 40. The pattern often runs in families, so you can expect to stop menstruating around the same time your mother, aunt or grandmother did, and at possibly the same rate as well.

The notorious "hot flashes" are believed to result from the impact of changing hormone levels on the temperature center of the brain—a kind of natural thermostat—located in the hypothalamus (the region that also monitors the menstrual cycle). About 75 percent of menopausal women experience these disquieting sensations which usually erupt about two years after the final period and often persist for another five. In some cases, however, they make their appearance before the monthly flow has stopped completely. The frequency, length and intensity of each "flash" can vary widely. Forty a day is typical for some, a scattered few for others; the episodes may last from a few seconds to 30 minutes, sometimes pervading the entire body. Any stimulus that raises body temperature can bring them on, including over-exertion, emotional outbursts, a poorly-ventilated room, heat, spicy food, caffeine and alcohol. Flashes are most often intense at night—and can result in bouts of insomnia—when the hypothalamus is especially sensitive to changes in heat.

An altered pattern of menstrual cycles is the usual first-alert signal that fertility is on the wane. (Ironically, late-in-life irregularity often sends worried women to their doctors, thinking they are pregnant.) During the climacteric, periods become increasingly unpredictable and erratic, with some cycles as short as three weeks, and others as long as six to 10 weeks apart. The flow may be markedly heavy, lingering, sometimes clotted, one month; scanty and short-lived the next. And more and more cycles will take place without any egg released by the ovary. For someone who has always been regular and who may have even relied on the "rhythm" method of birth control, this new inconsistency in the menstrual pattern may provoke a good deal of anxiety.

One diaphragm user in her late 40s was so unsettled

by repeated false alarms that she began finding excuses to avoid having sex or else repeatedly asked her husband to use a condom. This new "condition" for lovemaking caused him to lose his enthusiasm and his erection, and soon both partners were too troubled to derive much pleasure from sex at all. When they decided that a sexless marriage was an unhappy alternative, they sought the help of a therapist. The treatment was reassuringly simple: Once their physician informed them about natural menopausal changes and appropriate contraception, they were able to resume a more erotically satisfying life than ever. (See also the chapter on sex and the menstrual cycle.)

HOW MENOPAUSE HAPPENS

Why do periods become so problematic before menopause? And if fertility is declining, why is the bleeding often heavy or the cycles frequently shorter than usual?

The reasons are similar to those for menstrual irregularity in younger women: a lower than average hormone level means that the brain's pituitary gland is not receiving its customary shut-off signals or self-regulating feedback. Thus, in a *normal* cycle, when the primary female hormones, estrogen and progesterone, reach a certain high, the brain responds by reducing its output of FSH and LH (follicle-stimulating and luteinizing hormones) accordingly. (It is FSH and LH which cause the ovaries to release estrogen and progesterone in the first place.) But if both primary hormones are in chronically short supply, the pituitary will send out more FSH and LH, as if desperately trying to awaken the sluggish ovaries. When the latter fail to respond, the persistent pituitary pumps out even more of these chemical messengers, and so the vicious cycle continues. Eventually, the level of FSH may be as much as 13 times higher than normal in a premenopausal woman. The gross imbalance that results will soon show up as an altered cycle.

For example, with so much FSH around, the follicles tend to develop more rapidly than usual, though their total estrogen output may be very low. Even if an egg is released and a corpus luteum forms, the progesterone it secretes may also be inadequate. A faster follicle-ripening phase generally means that the cycle itself will be shortened by as much as four days or more.

As menopause nears, the ovaries stop producing eggs altogether, so progesterone is no longer secreted. This means that the uterine lining is now stimulated by estrogen alone. (Estrogen falls off less abruptly than progesterone and, as already mentioned, is still manufactured by part of the ovary or elsewhere in the body.) So the lining may continue to develop uninterruptedly until it finally outgrows its blood-vessel supply. At this point, it will begin to break down and shed, and the resulting period may be heavier than normal because of the extended tissue buildup. The flow may also be haphazard and prolonged as the overgrown uterine wall is cast off in sections at a time.

In some women, persistently low levels of estrogen in the absence of progesterone will produce only occasional spotting, which may be lingering but very light.

Ultimately, the ovaries' few remaining follicles are no longer sufficiently sensitive to the urgent signals from FSH and the estrogen level drops too far to build up any lining at all: Menstruation then ceases and the menopause is underway. To be on the safe side, some form of contraception should continue for about a year after the final period since an isolated egg or two may be released even months after the flow has stopped.

In some women, menopause gives very little warning—maybe two or three out-of-the-ordinary cycles—and then periods end rather suddenly. But more often, it is preceded by up to several years of menstrual unpredictability.

A late start at puberty may forecast an early menopause, though there is no clear-cut rule. Women who have had their Fallopian tubes tied or cut, or who have undergone hysterectomies with their ovaries left intact, are likely to experience menopause about two to three years earlier than average. Those who have never borne children tend to reach it *later* than normal.

Surgery, trauma or psychological shock and possibly nutritional factors can each delay or accelerate the process. And heredity seems to play a role as well: For example, orientals and caucasians of Northern European descent have a greater tendency to osteoporosis and vaginal atrophy than blacks or those of Mediterranean origin.

To determine that your climacteric has begun, your doctor may measure tissue samples from your vagina and uterus for signs of estrogen decline. Keep in mind that not every aspect of aging can be attributed to diminishing hormones. No direct link, for example, exists between loss of estrogen and facial wrinkles or crepey throats, joints and muscle pains or depression: Researchers have wryly observed that middle-aged men suffer comparable complaints! (Some researchers have noted that frequent, rapid mood surges may sometimes be caused by an *abrupt* drop in estrogen.) The three major problems that can be tied to altered hormones are hot flashes, vaginal changes and a higher risk of osteoporosis, the most serious affliction of all.

TROUBLE-FREE MENOPAUSE

Today, menopause is a far less traumatic passage than it was generations ago: The change-of-life blues are all but disappearing, thanks to greater medical know-how, tremendous lifestyle changes and healthier mental attitudes. Women are actively engaging their bodies and minds, remaining physically and sexually energetic, pursuing both familial and personal well-being. As a result, menopause looms far less threateningly than it once did to those whose lives were almost exclusively bound up with home and children: Then, the loss of fertility often signalled that their mission was essentially over.

No longer does menopause prophesy the end of vitality or fulfillment, but rather a new beginning that can usher in its own gratifications, sexual and otherwise. Perhaps most important of all, women today understand their bodies better and know how to seek appropriate medical help—often a problem for past generations when symptoms became unmanageable.

As with dysmenorrhea and PMS, any stress accompanying menopause is not a sign of mental aberration or emotional maladjustment, but is rather *biologically* based. In fact, medical doctors even 10 or 20 years ago were probably inclined to regard the menopause as the most physiological "female complaint." After all, they routinely prescribed estrogen to treat its troubling symptoms—and with apparent success.

During the 60s and 70s, already booming sales of estrogen replacement therapy (ERT) pills reached record highs. But then came the scary headlines. While women were curbing hot flashes an alarming number were falling victim to cancer of the uterine lining, a complication subsequently linked to the hormone supplement. Panic prevailed and the former "cure-all" was soon shunned by many doctors and patients alike.

Why cancer? The problem was simply that of replacing one hormone instead of two: As you have seen, menopause involves a decline in both hormones, estrogen *and* progesterone; when acting within the body these complement and counterbalance one another. Thus, estrogen *increases* the number of endometrial cells; then progesterone stops them from multiplying while it further matures and develops the uterine tissue so it can properly nourish an egg. Progesterone has a calming effect on the contracting muscles of the uterus (which is why inadequate amounts may contribute to the discomfort of PMS), changes the consistency of cervical mucus and "instructs" the hypothalamus to curb its production of LH.

While a rise in estrogen sets the stage for the endometrial buildup every month, the drop in progesterone is ultimately responsible for shedding it. Without this second regulating hormone, menstruation either does not take place or else only very erratically, marked by an abnormally heavy flow because so much uterine tissue has been allowed to form.

So consider what can happen if a menopausal woman is only given estrogen to ease her complaints: Without progesterone, it can lead to an unrelieved growth of tissue within the uterus. And this condition, called hyperplasia, is believed by some doctors to be the first step in a series of changes leading to uterine lining cancer.

It follows fairly logically (but since when is medicine always logical?) that estrogen per se is not the problem, but rather the failure to complete the replacement process by adding back progesterone as well. Since a woman's reproductive system is governed by both hormones, restoring only one to functioning levels may simply lead to an unnatural imbalance—and one consequence could be cancer. In fact, researchers have successfully tested this theory: Current evidence indicates that estrogen can be given with relative safety if (and only if) it is alternated cyclically with progesterone for at least 10 days—thus mimicking the normal cycle. In fact, women who do not receive this combined therapy may actually be the ones at increased risk of endometrial cancer and other diseases.

While effectively treating troubling physical symptoms, the estrogen/progesterone supplements have been shown to reduce cancer risk in women who receive post-menopausal hormone replacements. As you have seen, progesterone plays its protective role by countering the over-growth of endometrial tissue or hyperplasia, a possible prelude to malignancy associated with estrogen given alone. It also seems to buffer or control the absorption of estrogen by key "target" tissues. Estrogen overload is reportedly the major danger, so if progesterone is not administered properly or given for too short a period of time, it will not perform its crucial "blocking" action.

Alternating progesterone cyclically with estrogen may

cause a menstrual flow to occur each month: This "inconvenience" is presumably what led many physicians and patients to favor the giving of estrogen alone. But the monthly bleeding is a small price to pay for enhanced protection against serious disease. (Using the lowest dose of estrogen is much less likely to result in withdrawal bleeding, anyway.)

If a woman does take estrogen alone she may not be heightening her risk significantly if she takes the smallest possible doses for the least amount of time to be effective. But prolonged use of the hormone in isolation is another story: After two to four years, a woman's yearly chance of developing cancer is slightly increased over that of nonusers. The longer she takes estrogens, however, the greater the hazards. After five years' treatment or more, the incidence of tumors climbs from two to 10 times the norm in most studies. Remember, these statistics apply to estrogen administered in the *absence* of progesterone. When the two are taken cyclically together, some researchers have reported that the therapy may be *protective* against malignancy.

Other benefits of HRT: (Hormone Replacement Therapy)

• *Hot flashes respond rapidly to the treatment*, often subsiding within a week or two. No one knows for sure how the hormones work, but one theory is that they help stabilize the blood vessel system.

• *Vaginal atrophy can be relieved or reversed* in a matter of weeks or months: Declining hormone levels cause the vagina to shrink in length and width, and its substantial, fluid-rich layers of cells to thin out considerably. Blood flow is reduced, along with normally cleansing, anti-bacterial secretions. The result is a vagina susceptible to dryness, itching, irritation and infection—a condition called atrophic vaginitis. Intercourse can be extremely uncomfortable, even painful.

A woman's failure to lubricate adequately could have a devastating impact on her partner who may assume she is not responsive to *him*. In fact, a surprising number of older couples have brought themselves to therapists with sex problems related to one or another strictly biological fact of menopause. Once this is understood and the condition corrected, the "problems" promptly disappear.

Along with the natural muscle-toning effects of regular sex, HRT increases blood flow to the vaginal tissues, leaving them once again bathed in moisture, pink and youthful. Improvement is visible in a matter of weeks, depending on how advanced the atrophy was; severe cases may take a few months to "heal."

For women who were scared off by news of estrogen's adverse effects, physicians have often prescribed topical estrogen creams to restore lubrication. But recent studies show that these preparations carry the same degree of risk as the oral estrogens administered alone. The creams are effectively absorbed into the bloodstream and consistent use results in levels comparable to those sustained by the oral form of the hormone. So if you're using creams, be sure your doctor also administers progesterone to create a protective balance. (One advantage of the topical approach: It bypasses the liver and digestive tract and so is not broken down as the oral medications; delivery is more direct.)

• *Coronary disease risk may be reduced* (along with that of endometrial cancer): Almost everyone has heard that heart attacks are far more likely to strike men than women. However, after the menopause, a woman's apparent advantage disappears as her chance of developing atherosclerosis and other forms of coronary disease approaches that of a man. This circumstantial evidence points to estrogen as a probable protective factor. One study found that women whose ovaries were removed during hysterectomies before the age of 35 were at seven times the risk of heart attack for their age group.

Physicians and patients alike are already aware that birth control pills, which contain estrogen and progesterone and are given cylically, carrying warnings about possible cardiovascular complications. These include stroke, heightened blood pressure, clots and an increased likelihood of heart attack, particularly in smokers over 35. If this is so, why should HRT, which contains the very same hormones, be associated with a lower-than-average risk of heart disease?

For one thing, the dosages and formulas are very different. The amounts of estrogen used in oral contraceptives are up to a hundred times greater than those in HRT because they must be able to suppress ovulation and "shut down" the reproductive system—a biologically tall order. When the goal is only to restore flagging hormones to adequate levels, much lower dosages can be used. In addition, some birth control pills contain a form of progesterone derived from testosterone (called a progestogen) which has been implicated in blood vessel disorders, resulting in an increase in "bad" lipoproteins. But HRT commonly uses progestins, derived from natural progesterone, which have *not* been found similarly guilty.

Significantly, despite the endometrial cancer risk for estrogens used alone, studies of the effects of this replacement hormone (the low-dose kind) paint a favorable picture of longevity overall. For example, a five-year research project funded by the National Institutes of Health compared the medical histories of over 2,000 women between the ages of 40 and 69. The mortality rate of post-menopausal women on estrogen therapy was one-third that of women who had not taken hormone supplements! The women studied were grouped into three categories: those with normal reproductive function; those with a uterus removed, with or without one ovary; those with uterus and both ovaries removed. The result: Those who used no estrogen and had their uterus plus two ovaries removed had the highest death rate; estrogen users had the *lowest* mortality rates in all three categories.

One of the proposed reasons for estrogen's apparent life-extending effect is its connection with a rise in blood level of HDL—the so-called beneficial form of cholesterol (lipoprotein) that helps carry away deposits from vessels walls. As already discussed, progesterone essentially opposes or reverses the effects of estrogen on the body during the course of a cycle. Interestingly, the hormone replacement formulas which contain derivatives of natural progesterone (generically, medroxyprogesterone acetate) do *not* counteract the beneficial impact of natural estrogen on blood cholesterol. However, the progesterones that are derived from testosterones (such as those found in some kinds of the Pill) apparently do.

Probably the most compelling argument in favor of hormone replacement therapy is its apparent success in preventing or even reversing the dreaded, progressive and potentially life-threatening bone disease, osteoporosis, to which at least a quarter of post-menopausal women fall victim. (See p. 105 for details on osteoporosis and menopause.)

• *Some experts now speculate that women receiving replacement estrogen and progesterone may even have a reduced risk of breast cancer compared with non-treated women.* Several studies have already supported this theory and more investigation will be underway. Women who do develop breast cancer while taking hormone replacements have been reported to have better survival rates than those on no therapy at all as long as these tumors are estrogen dependent.

While the above presents a decidedly favorable picture of HRT, not every woman is an ideal candidate and there are those for whom the treatment may pose more risks than benefits. In addition, the very idea of taking hormone replacements may be objectionable to many, since the therapy itself suggests that menopause is somehow a deficiency disease rather than a normal biological process shared by all women. Rosetta Reitz puts it most thoughtfully in her book, *Menopause: A Positive Approach* (Penguin): ''The concept of replacement therapy is an affront to my sensibility. The implication is if I must have something replaced, it is because I have lost something, I am deficient in something. It is viewing . . . any menopausal woman from an entirely wrong perspective. The term 'replacement' in this context implies that I will be replaced to where I was when I was menstruating. Why? I don't want any more children . . . A woman's body cannot prepare itself for pregnancy for some 35 years and then stop doing so without her feeling the change. I accept that I'm a healthy woman whose body is changing. I have never felt more in control of my life than now, and I feel neither deficient nor diseased."[1]

The terminology *is* unfortunate—doctors would be wise to rethink the purpose and goals of hormone therapy and possibly coin a more appropriate way to describe it (or simply delete the word replacement). Such treatment is more like an *extension* of hormonal influence than a replacement, after all. Under no circumstances should it be considered lightly and every woman must carefully weigh her needs before making a decision. A number of alternative therapies are also possible for the more serious conditions relieved by replacement hormones.

A thorough medical history and physical exam are required before you can be a candidate for hormone therapy. The checkup should also include complete blood tests, Pap smear, breast examination, a baseline and possibly annual mammogram and an endometrial biopsy (prior to therapy and every year thereafter) to rule out the presence of any malignancy. (Estrogen can stimulate the growth of an already-existing, hormone-dependent tumor.)

As you return for periodic exams, dosages may be adjusted up or down, depending on side effects. For example, an excess of estrogen may promote swelling or tenderness of the breasts; too little or too much progesterone may bring on complaints similar to PMS. Frequently, through trial and error, you and your doctor can arrive at the safest, most effective level of medication.

Right now, new methods of estrogen delivery are being tested. One is a time-released pellet placed under the skin

[1] As quoted in *Harper's Bazaar*, November, 1979, "Menopause: The Estrogen Controversy."

which bypasses the stomach, intestines and liver, allowing estrogens to enter the bloodstream directly. This may permit lower hormone dosages to be used with equal potency, resulting in fewer side effects.

WHO SHOULD NOT USE HRT?

The following are currently considered contraindications to the use of hormone replacement therapy:
• Breast or endometrial cancer or other estrogen-dependent tumors
• History of blood clotting (thromboembolic) disorders
• Pregnancy
• Abnormal endometrial biopsy
• Undiagnosed vaginal bleeding
• Gallbladder disease
• Personal or family history of kidney, liver or heart disease
• Medication with DES or exposure to it before birth
There are a number of alternative treatments, including the following:
• *Bellergal S*, a medication consisting of phenobarbital (a sedative) and nervous sytem inhibitors, has been prescribed successfully for hot flashes, headaches, tension and other menopausal symptoms.
• *Clonidine*, a blood-pressure-lowering agent used to treat hypertension in the U.S. (it controls the dilation and contraction of blood vessel walls) has been approved by Canada at lower doses to alleviate hot flashes. The relatively mild possible side effects include fatigue, constipation, dry mouth, drowsiness and headache.
• *Depo-Provera* a form of progesterone derived from natural sources given in small doses by injection every three months, has been reported to relieve hot flashes in as many as half the women treated. (This is *not* to be confused with the controversial contraceptive which involves very high, sustained doses.)
• *Nutritional supplements*: Although no formal studies have been conducted, there is good clinical evidence that

certain nutritional supplements are successful in minimizing symptoms. These include 400 to 800 international units of vitamin D and up to 2 grams a day of calcium to prevent osteoporosis; at least 400 IUs of E a day to relieve hot flashes, maintain blood vessels and help restore vaginal moisture and elasticity; 50 to 200 mgs. of B6 for a healthy nervous system, along with adequate amounts of zinc, folic acid and vitamin B12.

Optimum nutrition resulting from sound eating habits and a proper use of supplements will maintain well-being and keep resistance high against any assault by a troubled menopause.

• *Vigorous exercise* strengthens bones and curbs depletion of calcium, thus delaying or preventing osteoporosis. One-half hour of exercise three times a week can help stave off bone loss and, in some cases, rebuild bone. It also mobilizes the estrogen stored in fatty tissues. Sustained aerobic workouts enhance cardiovascular fitness and stimulate the release of beta-endorphins which induce a euphoric "high" or sense of buoyant well-being. And, as the eight physician co-authors of *The Menopause Book* (Hawthorne-Elsevier/Dutton) observe, "An underexercised older woman ages more rapidly and more extensively, her bones lose calcium more quickly and become fragile, and her torso tends to bend forward as the spine softens and curves."

• *Diet*: It has been suggested that red meats, caffeine, excessive alcohol, refined white sugars and chocolate can all aggravate menopausal symptoms and perhaps should be avoided or kept to a minimum. A diet plentiful in fresh vegetables and fruits, grains, seafood, legumes and low-fat dairy products is advisable.

• *Over-the-Counter Lubricants*: Water-soluble, non-hormonal lubricants are available for vaginal dryness, including the old reliable, K-Y jelly.

• *Sex* (intercourse or self-stimulation) goes a long way toward maintaining vaginal tone, elasticity, healthy blood flow and the capacity to lubricate adequately.

103

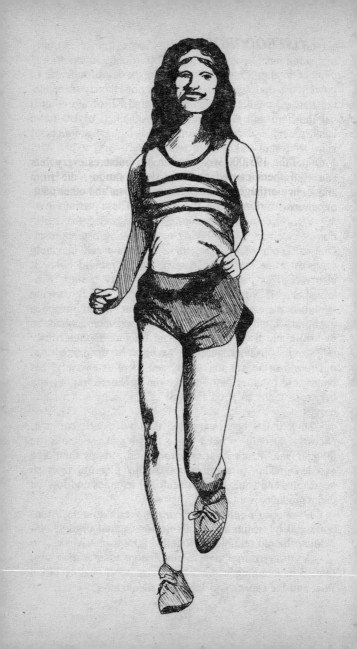

OSTEOPOROSIS

This is by far the most devastating possible outcome of menopause: Extensive bone loss entailing the risk of skeletal deformity and spontaneous fractures afflicts 25 percent of all post-menopausal Caucasian women. It strikes more commonly than rheumatoid arthritis, diabetes, heart disease, heart attacks, strokes or breast cancer. And it can *kill*. Many of the 195,000 women with hip fractures every year (most of them caused by bone deterioration), die from shock, hemorrhage, pneumonia, thrombosis and other complications resulting from the disease. These various hazards now constitute the twelfth leading cause of death in the United States. About another third of the victims require custodial care in nursing homes and remain severely disabled the rest of their lives.

Still another frequent and disfiguring result of osteoporosis is the collapse of one or more vertebrae, often resulting in significant loss of height, "dowager's hump," protruding stomach and distorted body proportions. Bones may be so brittle and fragile that they can fracture spontaneously as a result of everyday activities such as bending or lifting, opening a window, making a bed, even walking. Falls frequently result in breaks—or the breaks may actually occur first, precipitating the fall.

Bone tissue undergoes a constant cyclical process of building up and breaking down. Until about the early to mid-20s, the amount which is newly formed exceeds the tissue that is depleted or reabsorbed, resulting in a net gain of bone mass. Thereafter, however, the cycle reverses itself as the body begins to lose more bone than is replenished.

At menopause, the rate of bone breakdown increases dramatically, as the decline in estrogen impairs the body's capacity to use and absorb calcium. (Intestinal absorption of minerals in general also becomes less efficient with age.) The most rapid bone loss—up to three percent a year—occurs during the three years following cessation of monthly periods. Men lose bone mass with age, too, but far more gradually, and their skeleton is larger and denser to begin with. In addition, they do not undergo a sudden drop in hormone production that would affect the way their body controls bone development (and breakdown). After menopause, women lose bone at six times the rate of men, and so are far more likely victims of osteoporosis.

A sustained deficiency of calcium over several decades brought about by an inadequate diet, a sedentary lifestyle and hereditary factors may collectively set the stage for the disease. Obviously, some factors are simply beyond control: Women of Northern European, British, Chinese, and Japanese origin are at higher risk than those of North African, Mediterranean or Hispanic descent. (Bone density seems to be directly proportional to the amount of melanin or pigment in the skin.) The slight, slender, fair-skinned and light-haired are especially susceptible. And a relatively early menopause is another apparent risk: Since estrogen decline definitely accelerates bone loss, the earlier the hormone dropoff occurs, the more time a woman has to develop osteoporosis.

However, a number of risk factors *can* be controlled: low dietary intake of calcium and lack of exercise, especially, and perhaps smoking, heavy drinking, chronic stress and lack of sunshine. The body requires generous amounts of calcium because of its critical role in muscle, cardiac and nervous system function. If not enough of the mineral is available from dietary sources, the only storehouse left is the bone. Certain hormones will automatically stimulate the release of calcium from the skeleton to make up for the deficit. Thus, a chronic shortage of calcium over many years will literally chip away at the body's supporting structure.

How much calcium is enough? At least 800 to 1,000 mgs. a day before menopause and 1,200 to 1,400 mgs. during and after is the current recommendation. Pregnancy and lactation increase the daily requirement for younger women over 200 percent. To ensure an adequate intake, supplements (calcium carbonate, calcium lactate and calcium orotate are among the most readily absorbed of the formulas available) and plenty of calcium-rich foods such as dairy products, broccoli, turnip greens, salmon and sardines are advisable. During pregnancy, do not take any medicine, including vitamin and mineral supplements, without your obstetrician's knowledge.

But even if you are absorbing enough calcium, bear in mind that excesses of certain other foods may interfere with its absorption or hasten its excretion from the body. For example, it has been reported that an excess of protein may accelerate the loss of calcium from bones.

As with protein, too much phosphorus may sabotage calcium absorption—and Americans already get more than enough of it from meats, soft drinks, chemical additives, processed foods and breakfast cereals. In fact, most of us consume far more phosphorus than calcium—a ratio that should be reversed for any diet to be protective. In excessive amounts, bran fiber can bind calcium and other nutrients in the intestines, making them difficult to absorb; it also increases the rate at which all foods pass through the digestive tract, so fewer calories and minerals may be extracted. For overall health, fiber-rich grains are essential; however, avoid eating them *simultaneously* with calcium foods or supplements.

Nutritionists also caution about other *excesses* to be wary of: caffeine, tobacco, salt and alcohol. As for lifestyle, a steady onslaught of stress may hamper mineral absorption and increase the release of adrenal hormones which may encourage the loss of bone.

Regardless of which factors actually trigger the disease, consistent, vigorous exercise (in moderate, not excessive amounts) apparently helps prevent it and can retard the process by stimulating the growth of new bone. Even without a change of diet, physical activity has been shown to increase blood levels of calcium and to arrest bone deterioration. Muscle-contracting, limb-stretching exercises like jogging, bicycling, brisk walking, hiking and rowing are among the best choices because they put stress on bones, making them more durable and less subject to calcium resorption by the body.

The earlier you start exercising, watching your calcium intake and eliminating unnecessary stress, the better. The more bone mass you have developed (or salvaged) by age 35, the less vulnerable you will be to breakdowns and fractures once your estrogen supply diminishes.

As for the role of hormone replacements for osteoporosis, giving estrogen and progesterone at menopause can reduce the risk of vertebral collapse and fractures of hip and arm significantly if therapy lasts at least six years or longer. Even at the lowest doses available, estrogen can slow down the rate of bone breakdown and the loss of calcium via the kidneys. It also enhances the body's ability to absorb the minerals from food and supplements.

When hormone replacement therapy is administered cyclically at menopause the effects *are* dramatic—decreasing the rate of bone resorption and increasing calcium content. For women at risk, calcium/vitamin D therapy combined with hormone supplements can be a powerful preventive, more effective than the nutritional approach alone. Many physicians advise giving hormone replacements to small-boned, slim, sedentary women as a prophylactic measure.

Remember, only you and your doctor can decide whether you are a candidate for long-term estrogen/progesterone therapy. Note the contraindications listed on page 102 and consider whether the exercise and nutritional strategy would be protection enough.

I am a slender, sedentary, fair-skinned, light-eyed woman of Northern European descent with a family history of osteoporosis. Since that puts me in a high-risk category, I do intend to take hormone supplements as an added safeguard. (I may even begin an exercise program!) My co-author is an active woman of Mediterranean origin with no family history of the disease and would prefer the "natural" diet/exercise alternative before resorting to hormone therapy.

• *Fluoride Therapy*: Doctors at the Mayo Clinic in Rochester, Minnesota and Henry Ford Hospital in Detroit have successfully treated menopausal women with large doses of sodium fluoride plus calcium. Apparently, this combination stimulates bone-forming cells to manufacture new bone tissue faster than old cells are reabsorbed. Currently, researchers feel that the bone produced by this method is not as strong as normal growing bone tissue. Preliminary reports are guarded but promising. For example, in half the patients studied, the women showed very low fracture rates after one year of therapy. In addition, old fractures showed signs of healing and pain was markedly reduced. The possible drawbacks include rheumatic and gastrointestinal side effects.

• *Calcitonin*: This hormone, secreted by certain cells of the thyroid gland, enhances bone development and may slow down bone reabsorption or loss when given in combination with calcium and vitmain D. However, this is not a commonly used drug for the treatment or prevention of post-menopausal osteoporosis.

Remember, bone loss, while preventable, is largely irreversible—which means you should take the earliest steps to ensure healthy bones. Early diagnosis (not usually possible in a routine physical exam) is also desirable. Unfortunately, osteoporosis is silent and insidious— a woman often loses a considerable amount of bone mass before she has any symptoms or seeks medical help.

Some experts believe that low back pain and certain forms of periodontal disease are preliminary warning signs. Today, two sophisticated, expensive clinical tools, the CAT scan and photon (light) absorption can detect small changes in bone mass years before full-blown disease sets in. Right now, neither technique is widely available, but their screening abilities look promising, especially for women who are at high risk for osteoporosis.

Chapter 6

UPDATE: TOXIC
SHOCK SYNDROME

During the spring and summer of 1980, a "new" disease—swift in its onset and often deadly—was making headlines almost daily. Nearly all its victims were young, seemingly healthy menstruating women who were suddenly stricken with a cluster of baffling symptoms: dizziness, chills, fever that hovered near 104°, vomiting, diarrhea, a scaly, sunburn-like rash on the palms and soles, muscle aches, dangerously low blood pressure, kidney or liver failure, even shock. Most telling of all, 95 percent of those who succumbed were users of tampons. The highest risk seemed to involve wearers of the latest, most comfortable super-absorbent variety (of which the most popular brand at the time was *Rely* by Procter & Gamble).

Before this decade, most people had never heard of the mysterious malady, called toxic shock syndrome (TSS). Certainly, tampons, innocuous products by anyone's standards, had been in use since the mid-1930s. And, no more menacing, the bacterium (staphylococcus aureus) responsible for the illness had been around a long time as well: Whence their new association with a life-threatening disease?

Now that several years have passed, why has the early furor all but disappeared? Is the syndrome still flourishing, but no longer reported simply because novelty and interest have waned? And, if so, are tampon wearers still at risk?

Reports of any new, abruptly attacking disease are always terrifying because medical science seems to be caught off guard—lacking a basic understanding of its origins and the proper remedies by which to treat it. The body's defenses are confronted with an unaccustomed challenge and may simply not be able to control it. However, several years of research have unraveled some of the mysteries of toxic shock, though much remains to be explored. Here is what scientists know to date:

Millions of women and men harbor the syndrome-triggering bacterium, staph aureus, a common resident of the skin, mucous membranes of the nose and throat, vaginal wall and other areas. The organism thrives in the vaginas of about five to 10 percent of women; a large percentage carry the bacterium in the vulva or outer, lip-like surface of the vagina. However, the majority of us do *not* contract toxic shock either because we don't carry the form of staph aureus that results in the disease or because we have antibodies that specifically ward it off.

Actually, TSS has been recognized as a disorder since 1927, though its incidence was so uncommon as to be virtually invisible from public view. Then, sometime in the late 1970s, just as superabsorbent tampons came on the market, the disease came out of hiding—dramatically. Twelve cases, all involving tampon wearers, were brought to the attention of the Centers for Disease Control (CDC) in Atlanta, all with markedly similar and potentially fatal complaints. As a result—and virtually overnight—millions of menstruating women stopped using tampons altogether and started buying sanitary napkins until the damning circumstantial evidence could be explained.

In those women who were susceptible because of low resistance and/or because they already carried the organism intervaginally, the tampons may have created an environment favorable to the growth of what turned out to be a new, more troubling strain of staph aureus. Super absorbent tampons generally left in the vagina for long periods of time may allow this toxin-releasing staph aureus to reproduce rapidly. Under the right conditions, the bacterium produces a toxin that wreaks havoc on many areas of the body by overpowering the immune system and blocking the liver from performing its normal detoxifying functions.

The synthetic fibers from which the tampons are made are also believed to create imperceptible lacerations—and sometimes microscopic ulcers—in the vaginal wall, through which the toxins can pass easily into the bloodstream. In addition, superabsorbency may dry out the normally protective fluids in the vagina's mucous membrane, thus leaving it more vulnerable to irritations or infection—and penetration by the toxin. The tampons themselves do *not* harbor the substance; rather, their presence may serve as a catalyst for the disease to develop in a small percentage of women.

Very quickly, the syndrome moved up from the status of very rare to rare. The incidence, based on statistics compiled by the Minnesota State Health Department, is estimated to be about seven to 15 out of 100,000 annually, hardly the widespread menace that more than a few early sensational stories suggested. Still, on a nationwide basis, that rate should translate roughly into 4,500 cases every year, although (apparently) only a percentage of these cases have been officially reported. According to Minnesota investigators, the disease remained as prevalent as ever even after the notorious *Rely* was pulled off supermarket shelves—probably at least in part because other similarly made, though less publicized, products filled the resulting vacuum.

When the immune system in certain individuals is already ill-equipped to combat toxic shock and is overwhelmed by the disease, normally "friendly" microbes throughout the body are allowed to multiply unimpeded, with possibly devastating impact. This (and the systemic effects of the toxin) accounts for the grouping of symptoms that characterizes TSS—the liver and kidney damage, the decline in the number of blood platelets, the precipitous drop in blood pressure, the gastrointestinal problems and shock. The now unfettered bacteria in these well-scattered sites produce a highly virulent substance called endotoxin, which is responsible for the range of serious complaints.

Not all toxic shock is deadly; in fact, most of the cases are highly treatable with a relatively short hospital stay if spotted early enough (intravenous fluids to maintain blood pressure and appropriate antibiotics are part of the therapy). And a number of patients who have some (partial) built-in immunity develop milder forms of the disease.

Although associated automatically with tampons and menstruating women, toxic shock can strike individuals of either sex at any age, according to a recent news release from *The American Medical Association*. One case reported in early 1983 involved a 30-year-old man, for example, who suffered the usual array of alarming symptoms. Sure enough, staph aureus bacteria were present—cultured from lesions of shingles or "herpes zoster" on the young man's back. The patient's doctor reports that the number of bacteria on the skin lesions could not have been large, which means that the toxin they produced must have been very powerful.

According to Dr. Arthur L. Reingold, M.D., of the Centers for Disease Control, scientists now know that the syndrome can afflict a wide variety of patients, children included. About 15 percent of cases currently involve surgical wound infections; infected burns, scratches and insect bites; septic abortion; post-partum infection and a number of other conditions *unrelated* to menstruation and tampon use.

A few cases involved women who resorted to sea sponges or diaphragms to collect menstrual fluid; presumably, these had the same skin-lacerating impact on the vaginal wall as the synthetic-fibered tampons. Recently, developers of the new contraceptive vaginal sponge, *Today*, have begun investigating whether the product, which can be worn for as long as 24 hours, will promote growth of the toxic-shock producing organism. Certainly the risk of toxic shock syndrome increases when *anything* is left in the vagina for too long a period of time. (See also p. 135).

The same staph infection can enter through any break in the skin and give rise to a number of serious illnesses *aside* from TSS, such as infection of the heart valves, for example. While the new deviant bacterial strain is actually believed to be in its waning days, it is apparently being replaced by an equally potent toxin-producer, another reason the disease itself may not have abated.

If it *is* true that incidence of the disease has not significantly declined since 1980 (more documentation is needed to prove this beyond a doubt) what is the latest verdict on tampon use? How can you reduce your risks?

Based on recommendations from the American College of Obstetricians and Gynecologists: Be sure to change tampons at least every four to six hours and wear napkins on alternating days. Or else wear tampons only while you're flowing heavily; switch to napkins for lighter days and nighttime. Avoid the superabsorbent brands which may cause cuts or lacerations in the vaginal wall through which already-existing bacteria could enter. Since the disease reportedly has a 30 to 40 percent recurrence rate, women who have been treated for toxic shock are advised to avoid tampon use indefinitely. (Clearly, people who contract the disease more than once have not been able to develop the proper arsenal of antibodies to fight it after their first exposure.)

Now a simple blood test (radioimmunassay) can determine whether you are at risk for toxic shock by checking for the presence of specific antibodies that can fight the virulent toxins. Unlike most diagnostic tests, it's the *absence* of a reaction that is significant. About 95 percent of normal adults have circulating antibodies to the toxin, but only a few patients with acute toxic shock syndrome have been found with any detectable ''defenses.''

The availability of such a lab test to decide susceptibility to the syndrome will be able to identify those women—

the vast majority—who have nothing to fear from using tampons. Those whose blood samples contain no noticeable antibodies can then be advised by their doctors to discontinue or modify tampon use according to current cautions and to be on the alert for symptoms of the disease during a menstrual period.

Keep in mind that sanitary napkins are now vastly improved—many of them far thinner and more compressed than the traditional pads, but equally absorbent; they are also self-adhesive, attaching easily to an undergarment of any material. Gone are the days of bulky, cumbersome, chafing pads with their attendant paraphernalia of elastic belts, pins, metal hoods and straps.

For days of heaviest flow, super or maxi-pads or maxi-shields—many constructed to be as unobtrusive as possible without compromising (external) absorbency—may be worn as an alternative to tampons. Scented or deodorant varieties of each are available. Smaller "mini" pads provide protection on light-flow or tapering-off days, or can be used together with tampons when the flow is heavy.

Besides following the current guidelines, remember to cleanse the vulva (outer skin of vagina) thoroughly at least twice a day while menstruating and always wash hands well, too, before inserting a tampon or any contraceptive device.

Contrary to the biblical description, menstruation is *not* "unclean," but rather visible evidence that a natural internal cleansing of the uterus is taking place. Menstrual fluid and perspiration themselves have a minimal odor, if any, unless allowed to remain on the skin surface and exposed to air and bacteria; that's why simple soap-and-water showering or bathing is the most effective way of keeping the body odor-free at this time.

One caution: the practice of vaginal douching has become subject to increasing disfavor among physicians, and deservedly so. For example, a relationship between frequent, vigorous douching and salpingitis or pelvic inflammation has been established. Douching has also been linked to dryness and irritation of vaginal membranes.

Chapter 7

SEX AND THE MENSTRUAL CYCLE

Are we cyclically programmed to be sexier at certain times of the month than at others? Are we easily arousable when we are most fertile?

A number of surveys have reported that women are especially interested in sex at two crucial moments in the cycle—ovulation (at about the midpoint) and just before menstruation. One study, for example, showed that the level of erotic desire and activity in women increased about 25 percent around the time of ovulation, but not in those who were on the Pill (and who were thus not ovulating at all).

To account for this from a strictly biological view: at ovulation, a newly-ripened egg is released from its follicle nest and begins to make its four-day journey to the Fallopian tubes where it may rendezvous with a sperm cell. That means if you have intercourse before, during or not long after this time, your chances of becoming pregnant are fairly good. If nature wanted to ensure the continuation of the species, she could not have chosen a more appropriate time to awaken sexual interest.

As estrogen reaches its all-time high, the surge of progesterone at mid-cycle is accompanied by a peak in the production of testosterone from a woman's adrenal glands. And it is this male hormone that makes the nerve endings in her clitoris more sensitive to touch and heightens her sex drive.

"At no other time in the cycle do these three hormones coincide in her in the same way," observe Joe Durden-Smith and Diane Desimone, authors of the provocative new book, *Sex And The Brain* (Arbor House). "Only at ovulation do they conspire to give her this unique readiness for sex, as well as an enhancement of her immune system and three of her senses: sight, taste and smell." This may well be a holdover from the old mechanism that makes female primates receptive at one point in their cycle, and it is still *part* of our evolutionary program today, the authors suggest.

Just before or during the menstrual period, hormone levels have sharply dropped and a new egg-containing follicle has not yet begun developing. So, if the studies are any accurate index, women are just as erotically inclined when fertility is at its lowest, or when they are least worried about becoming pregnant. But more likely, any possible increase in libido at this point is the result of the natural swelling and congestion of uterine and vaginal tissue just before the flow that is physically arousing.

Despite our highly evolved social rituals and cultural sophistication, sexuality is not completely independent of biological forces. However, the problem with searching for and even establishing connections between hormone levels and shifting erotic moods is that it leaves out what motivates us to engage in sex more than anything else—mental and emotional influences. We are largely cerebral beings and the head is the most erogenous zone of all. We are potentially responsive (or not) any time during our cycle, depending on a host of environmental variables. This continual sexual "availability"—and apparent freedom from strictly cylical urges—is what distinguishes us from all other female members of the animal kingdom! The fact that men and women can and seek to "mate" at any time during the monthly cycle is considered by some scientists to be a primary factor in the evolution of human societies—making possible and desirable the realities of erotic *love* and enduring family bonds.

118

In addition, some studies purporting to relate the monthly cycle to sexual desire show conflicting or inconclusive findings. Human sexuality is, after all, a good deal more complicated than even the already intricate ebb and flow of hormones would suggest.

SEX DURING MENSTRUATION?

One survey, recently referred to in *Medical Aspects of Human Sexuality* suggests that intercourse during mensutation is less common than at any other time—not a surprising finding. Thus, when asked whether they desired sex or not, more women said "yes" during their non-menstruating days.

This does not necessarily mean that interest in lovemaking wanes when the flow appears: Cultural conditioning, esthetic aversion, a partner's objection or religious restraints may be powerful inhibitors. The possible discomfort of premenstrual symptoms or dysmenorrhea may also dampen anyone's mood for sexual pleasure. Interestingly, Masters and Johnson found that a number of women reported masturbating at or just before the onset of menstruation in order to reach orgasm and thus find relief from either distressing or sexually arousing pelvic congestion.

Is it possible to become pregnant during a period? Women rarely conceive at the beginning of a new cycle since a mature follicle has not yet had time to develop and release an egg destined for the uterus. (Nor is the uterus, which is in the process of shedding or breaking down, prepared to support a fertilized egg.) However, it's possible for some spotting or even bleeding to occur at the time of ovulation. If a woman should mistake this for the start of a menstrual period and have intercourse without contraception, she could conceive.

If a woman ovulates early—say, six or seven days into her cycle instead of the usual 12 to 14—and has a relatively short interval between periods, she may become pregnant if she has sex during menstruation since a sperm cell can live in the genital tract for about 72 hours as it awaits an approaching egg. Pregnancy is also possible if menstrual bleeding is prolonged because of some irregularity; or if a woman continues to spot at some other time in her cycle, mistakes this for menstruation and proceeds to have unprotected intercourse.

If you object to sex during your periods for whatever reason, remember that wearing a diaphragm can stop the flow temporarily. Or, strategic use of the Pill can prevent menstruation at inopportune times, such as a vacation or honeymoon. You can simply stay on the oral contraceptive beyond the usual period of three weeks to cover the entire time you are away. At the end of this interval, discontinuing the hormones will bring on withdrawal bleeding. For example, if a marriage ceremony is scheduled three weeks from the date that a Pill cycle is set to begin, instead of stopping the pills at the end of three weeks, continue taking them for four or five weeks to prevent and delay the onset of bleeding.

SEX AND MENARCHE

Menarche is the main event of puberty, the visible, irrevocable proof of potential fertility and sexual awakening. Almost every woman can recall vividly the details of her very first period—where she was, with whom, what she was doing at the time, how she felt about it. Even in our jaded, rational age, it still inspires awe or delight or fear or some unnamable mix of feelings; it's still a momentous passage.

If you have a daughter, your attitudes about menstruation and your body will greatly influence the shaping of her own. The best time to start discussing the forthcoming period is when she is about nine or 10. Watch for the early signs of physical maturity such as breast development, the appearance of pubic or underarm hair—usually preludes to menstruation. Let her know what kinds of changes to expect, that monthly bleeding is a natural, healthy process, not an illness or disability. The more informed she is about her body, the better prepared she will be to take charge of her own health—and this awareness cannot begin too soon. Ideally, a son or husband should participate in these discussions as well. No man should be excluded from the realities of menstruation, as if it were a shameful secret or damaging to some ideal image of womanhood. By knowing the facts, he will have a healthy respect for female biochemistry, without viewing it with inappropriate awe, anxiety or distaste.

Before the first menstrual period, the onrush of maturing hormones is already stirring intense, unaccustomed, often overwhelming drives and feelings; these need to be identified and acknowledged. As your daughter becomes biologically ready for sex, peer pressures to "experiment" may heighten the existing turmoil. When it does occur, menarche is a logical time to explore (and share) sexual feelings, values, pleasures, fears; the realities of fertility and contraception. (See pages 126 for an update on birth control methods.)

Are teenage girls as sexually sophisticated as current impressions suggest? The rising rate of pregnancies among this age group would seem to argue yes. However, physicians report that a fair number of young women have admitted to engaging in sex because "everyone else" seems to be doing it or because their boyfriends are persuasive. They often say they agree for fear of being excluded socially or rejected by a current partner. For this reason, it is especially important to note that many "popular" and well-adjusted girls are not sexually active— and that giving in to pressure is as restrictive and confining as the unquestioned values of earlier times. You don't have to have sex if you don't want to; imitating others' behavior is hardly the way to liberation.

According to Dr. Ezra Davidson, professor and chairman of obstetrics and gynecology at New York University Medical Center, as quoted in a recent article/panel discussion in *Sexual Medicine Today*, "Abstinence is a real alternative:

What is not emphasized enough is the large number of young people who are *not* sexually involved," and this is creating a distorted, exaggerated view. Adolescents need to be aware of the choices and decisions they have to make when they are being "strong-armed" by their peers to participate in sexual activity, Dr. Davidson adds. "They need to develop *values* (preferably through discussion with parents or other adults) so they know how they are going to behave *before* the pressures confront them."

As for fertility at menarche: Just as the premenopausal years of a woman's reproductive life are marked by increasingly irregular, anovulatory periods because of a gradual loss of estrogen, so, too, a girl's earliest menstruating years—when hormones have not yet reached their peak or proper balance—are not typically highlighted by ovulatory, fertile cycles. In one Finnish study of 200 girls, between 55 and 80 percent of the menstrual cycles were without ovulation within the first two years of menarche. By five years after the first period, the number had dropped to 20 percent. However, a tendency to infertile cycles does not mean that ovulation cannot or will not occur during a given month. So, unless she wants to conceive, no menstruating women at any age should have intercourse without contraception.

SEX AT MENOPAUSE

Few women ultimately regret the loss of their fertility, and most of them have ample time to adjust to the idea—only rarely does menstruation end abruptly. However, some do interpret this midlife slide in hormones as a sign of diminishing femininity, youth or sexual attractiveness—and the attitude can become a self-fulfilling prophecy.

Linda K. studied herself in the mirror and noted the changes. Hairs sprouting from her chin, deeper wrinkles near the eyes and mouth, more fat around her middle. And, yes, there was one other change she was almost too embarrassed to mention to her doctor: After 37 years of marriage, she and her husband were no longer having sex.

One problem was her lowered self-esteem—she no longer felt desirable or sensual because of all her bodily changes, and so she began avoiding intercourse, feigning fatigue or finding excuses. But the other reason was more immediate, physical: sex had simply become too painful. As described in the chapter on menopause, the once thick and supple tissues lining her vagina had become thin, dry and irritated because less estrogen was available to nourish them. Also, she noticed she was less sensitive to touch, especially around her breasts—her skin felt numb and tingling. As for her husband, it was no longer as easy for him to have or sustain an erection—and she began to think that she was really to blame, that he had become less interested in their relationship.

Here is a woman experiencing two kinds of problems, both very real and mutually reinforcing. The menopausal decline in estrogen can result in vaginal atrophy—a loss of blood supply and lubricating fluids in the genital area, causing tissue to shrink, dry out and lose its elasticity. Other possible estrogen-related changes are altered sensitivity in the clitoris and breasts, cramping after orgasm and a burning sensation upon urination after intercourse. If they are seriously disrupting your sexual enjoyment, these conditions can be remedied by minimal, short-term doses of hormone replacement therapy (estrogen alternated with progesterone in a cyclical pattern) or, possibly, by some of the alternative approaches also featured in Chapter 5.

This woman is also suffering from a loss of self-esteem and sexual confidence: Accepting the myth that midlife is a time of deterioration and loss, rather than renewal and growth; that sexual energies diminish with the end of fertility, she convinces herself that she is no longer desirable and assumes that her husband secretly agrees, under the guise of a sexual "problem." She resigns herself to the "inevitable" instead of seeking solutions. But a vicious cycle is at work: By avoiding lovemaking altogether, she may be aggravating the very vaginal complaint that has made sex so uncomfortable in the first place.

Recently, researchers at the Rutgers University Medical School reported in the *Journal of the American Medical Association* that post-menopausal women who remain sexually active (and that includes self-stimulation) undergo significantly less vaginal deterioration than those of the same age group who abstain or have sex infrequently. The study measured differences in the depth, resilience, health of mucous membranes, cell blood supply and other factors, and concluded that the results lent "some support for the adage 'use it or lose it.' " (The Rutgers study group has defined sexually active women as those who engage in intercourse at least three times a month, and inactive women as those whose frequency is less than 10 times a year. Other studies have found that masturbation is just as effective for keeping the vagina in peak condition.)

The research also supports recent findings that androgens (the male hormones testosterone and androstenedione) are the primary catalysts for a woman's sex drive. And it shows, too, that women who are less sexually involved after menopause have decreased levels of androgens along with greater signs of vaginal atrophy.

While vaginal muscle and tissue changes may reduce the intensity of orgasmic contractions and the amount of lubrication during intercourse, a woman whose sex life continues can maintain normal levels of pleasure. It has been observed that the more the body gets used to being aroused and having orgasmic release, the easier it becomes to respond. The Kegel exercises, recommended for after childbirth, also help keep vaginal tissues toned and youthful. These involve tensing the pubococcygeous muscle (the one that controls urine flow) for one second, then relaxing it for one. The exercises can be done anywhere, and many doctors advise a total of about 100 to 200 a day.

While so many women fear a loss of libido as estrogen levels decline with age, often just the opposite occurs—the hormonal drop actually *intensifies* desire. Why? Testosterone, the male hormone present in both sexes, is chiefly responsible for fueling sexual arousal in women and men. With less estrogen around to "compete" with testosterone after menopause, the male hormone's effects as an erotic stimulant become more pronounced than ever.

For many women at menopause, release from the fear of pregnancy generates a new appetite for sex. One 50-year-old woman admitted that intercourse for her was always accompanied by what she calls "the anxiety of uncertainty" —meaning less-than-foolproof birth control: "I consider the end of menstruation the beginning of a new life!"

Other women report that the proverbial and dreaded "empty nest" becomes an unexpectedly delightful love nest as they and their husbands suddenly become a couple again, with the house all to themselves, freed from the cares and distractions of childrearing. "My husband and I can stay in bed late on Saturday mornings, have dinner out more often, make love when or wherever we want," one woman explains. "Just being alone together again reminds us of the time when we were first married—and our sex life has picked up accordingly!"

After 40, a woman's relationship can be enhanced by a physiological slowdown in her partner as well: What might loom as a worrisome decline or a withdrawal of interest to some may prove very desirable to others. An older man has less of a need to ejaculate, takes longer or more direct stimulation to have an erection—and that means his needs and timing are better synchronized with those of his wife. He can sustain and enjoy foreplay more than ever, which can heighten sexual pleasure for both.

Only if male or female bodily changes are *misinterpreted* will they result in conflict. Thus, if a woman takes longer or fails to lubricate, her partner may blame himself for not adequately arousing her. So he may try harder to make her respond, turning sex into an assignment with a specific goal—and nothing can be more inhibiting. Both become anxious spectators, waiting for her to "come around." Similarly, if a woman, already haunted by self-doubt,

125

fearful of losing her vigor and youth, believes her husband's slower sexual reflexes mean he finds her unattractive, she may feel resentment or a loss of self-worth, which can only impair her ability to respond and experience pleasure. Or, if he interprets his slower tempo as proof of declining potency, the results could be equally devastating.

The key is to know your body, to become aware of the ways it will change and why so you can adapt to them, sexually and otherwise. Just knowing what menopause entails and the natural, physiological reasons for midlife shifts in timing or response can spare you much confusion and anxiety. Simply sharing concerns and discussing bodily changes can make them seem less overpowering. If you recognize that what is happening is normal, you can even discover new joys, become more sexually inventive: You may find that "taking longer" allows you to savor lovemaking more, both its minor delicious moments and the major ones. And with intercourse changing its pattern, you might choose to broaden your repertoire with massage or oral sex. If you and your partner can continue to communicate openly about sexual needs, there is no reason why you should not remain vibrant and sensual to the end of your life.

CONTRACEPTION UPDATE: FROM MENARCHE TO MENOPAUSE

The ideal solution to birth control continues to elude us, but today the range of choice is enormous—what some doctors have referred to as a "cornucopia" of contraceptive possibilities. There is literally a method for everyone, to accommodate every need and circumstance. How you choose is a highly individual matter and your preferences may change along with your priorities or state of health throughout your childbearing years. But in any case, safety, effectiveness and convenience should be No. 1 considerations. Here is a brief roundup, including current pros and cons:

The Pill

In recent years, following a spate of scary headlines, there has been a marked decline in the use of oral contraceptives (OCs). However, they still remain the most reliable, effective and popular alternative for women under 35—and the news right now should be enough to spur a mini-revival of the Pill. (The drop in Pill use has occurred primarily among teenagers and women in their early 20s, ironically the least vulnerable of any group to its health risks. In fact, teenagers are five times more likely to die of pregnancy-related causes than of complications resulting from the Pill.)

Women with the highest possibility of complication are those predisposed to blood clotting, strokes, liver, heart disease, estrogen-dependent cancers and those over the age of 35. Also, anyone who takes the Pill and smokes faces higher odds of falling victim to heart attack and stroke than non-smoking Pill users. Despite this, an estimated 85 percent of women are good candidates.

How it works: The Pill contains high enough levels of synthetic estrogen and progesterone to "fool" the body into a perennially "pregnant" state, hormonally speaking, thus curbing the release of its own natural hormones from the hypothalamus and pituitary. This prevents ovulation or the release of an egg from an ovarian follicle and, in effect, closes down the normal menstrual cycle. The progesterone in the Pill also thickens the cervical mucus, making it impenetrable to sperm. Because the hormones in the Pill, mimicking those of the body, stimulate the growth of the endometrium, bleeding occurs during the fourth week of every month when a woman has a Pill-free interval (a kind of artificial menstruation).

One 24-year-old patient started out with a low-dose oral contraceptive, but was bothered by repeated episodes of breakthrough bleeding. This is a temporary reaction to the formula, which a doctor can alleviate by administering a slightly higher dose of estrogen for a short period of time if the bleeding doesn't stop on its own. Mini-Pills containing only progesterone are often prescribed for women with conditions that may be aggravated by estrogen—hypertension, migraines, varicose veins. These work by thickening the cervical mucus and interfering with the buildup of the uterine lining to prevent a fertilized egg from implanting there.

Often, symptoms resulting from the Pill are the result of too much or too little estrogen, progesterone or both, depending on the dosage prescribed for you: for example, nausea, headache, vomiting, weight gain, acne, brown blotches on the skin, breast tenderness, bloating. These sometimes can be minimized or eliminated by readjusting the formula. That's why an ongoing dialogue between you and your doctor spelling out your day-to-day response to the contraceptive is crucial to arriving at the balance of hormones which works best for you. Women on the Pill also have heightened needs of certain nutrients, especially vitamins of the B complex group (see Chapter 8.)

When you go off the Pill and wish to become pregnant you should use an alternate method for three or four months after to be certain there are no harmful effects on the fetus from the lingering effects of the drug. Some women may find they fail to menstruate after discontinuing the Pill, a condition called Post-Pill amenorrhea which can last a number of months. This phenomenon is temporary except in rare cases. If a woman does not return to normal periods within a year and wishes to conceive, a fertility drug called Clomid, which acts on the pituitary in a similar way as estrogen, can reactivate her cycle by stimulating the proper ratio and release of the two key menstrual hormones, FSH and LH.

Most recently, it has been found that the Pill may have some advantages beyond preventing pregnancy. Users are reportedly less likely to develop endometrial and ovarian cancer since incessant ovulation is associated with an increased risk. Also, by reducing the number of days of the menstrual flow, it prevents bacteria from entering the Fallopian tubes and may therefore protect against sexually transmitted diseases. And, the fact that estrogen—a major component of most OCs—stimulates both normal and malignant breast tissue does not mean it causes breast cancer. In fact, the Pill has been associated with a decreased likelihood of benign or fibrocystic breast disease and has *not* been linked with a heightened risk of breast cancer.

Oral contraceptive users have a 40 percent lower chance of contracting pelvic inflammatory disease (PID) than women using no birth control at all. A lower-than-average incidence of VD, rheumatoid arthritis and menstrual cramps has been reported among Pill users as well.

Note: Report to your doctor any such symptoms as the following: pains in the leg, chest, abdomen, severe headaches, dizziness, vision changes or numbness in any part of the body. Aside from the women mentioned above who should definitely not consider the Pill, there are those for whom it may not be advisable for other than short-term use or except during special circumstances. These include women with migraine headaches, diabetes or pre-diabetes (the mini-Pill is a possible alternative in this case), undiagnosed vaginal bleeding, a history of irregular or anovulatory cycles, severe depression, chest pain, asthma, epilepsy or hypertension. Other relative contraindications are varicose veins, uterine fibroids (consider the mini-Pill), systemic diseases such as thyroid disorders, multiple sclerosis, lupus, etc., obesity, heavy smoking and known elevated serum triglycerides.

Anyone considering oral contraceptives should discuss her medical history carefully with her doctor, as well as undergo a complete gynecological checkup.

The IUD

Its rate of effectiveness is second only to that of the Pill and an estimated 10 to 12 percent of American women (2.5 to 3 million) practicing birth control are wearing them. As with the Pill, some of the drawbacks have been widely publicized: For example, studies have shown that users are three to five times more likely to develop pelvic inflammatory diseases (PID)—inflammation of the Fallopian tubes, uterus or ovary which may cause ectopic pregnancy (a fetus growing outside the uterus) or even sterility—than non-users; the chances are greatest for women 25 and under and those with multiple sexual partners. The *length* of time an IUD remains in the uterus so far has not been connected with pelvic infection, but insertion or reinsertion has been associated with an increased risk. (The symptoms of PID include unusual discharge, abdominal or pelvic pain, fever and painful intercourse.)

Other possible complications include displacement or expulsion during menstruation, cramping and heavy menstrual bleeding (most likely during the first six months after insertion), implantation within the uterine wall and very rarely, perforation of the uterus. Also, should you become pregnant while the device is in place, you run a higher-than-normal risk of septic abortion.

How it works: Available in a variety of shapes, sizes and materials, the IUD is implanted by a physician through the cervical canal; threads attached to the small device extend outside the cervix to allow the wearer to check periodically that the IUD is properly placed. (Slippage is relatively rare.) The presence of an IUD, a foreign body in the uterus, is believed to create an inflammation which prevents a fertilized egg from implanting in the uterine wall. It may also do its job by hampering movement of sperm through the uterus as well as the egg's transit through the Fallopian tubes.

Like the Pill, the IUD is unobtrusive (it does not interfere with sexual spontaneity) and highly effective. The best time to have one inserted is during your period, to make sure you aren't pregnant while wearing the device. Once in place, it's important to feel for the retrieval thread at regular intervals to determine that the IUD is still in position.

For women with a tendency to dysmenorrhea or already heavy periods, the IUD may not be a desirable choice. However, one small-sized variety called the progestasert contains enough progesterone to counteract such effects in some users. Selection of IUD type should depend on your menstrual history, the size of your uterus and childbearing history, among other considerations. Generally, physicians are not inclined to regard the IUD as a first-choice contraceptive for women who have not borne children.

Who should not wear an IUD; women with abnormal Pap smears, blood clotting disorders, a history of pelvic inflammation or ectopic pregnancy. Also, those with anemia, severe menstrual problems, fibroid tumors or endometriosis are advised to choose another form of contraception. Report any chills, fever, abdominal pains, unexplained bleeding or pain during intercourse to your doctor since any one of these can signal problems with the IUD.

The Diaphragm and other Barrier Methods

The percentage of women using barrier methods of contraception nearly tripled between 1973 and 1979 and the numbers probably reflect former Pill and IUD users, says Dr. Enayat Elahi, medical director of Planned Parenthood in New York City. There are no serious side effects associated with the diaphragm or condom and such "barrier" methods may protect against the agents of sexually transmitted diseases.

All barrier contraceptives work, as their name suggests, by placing either a physical or chemical obstacle between the sperm and the egg. A flexible, dome-shaped (round or oval) rubber cup stretched around a steel spring, the diaphragm is inserted into the vagina to cover the opening of the cervix. For maximum protection, it is coated with a spermicidal cream or jelly, preferably inside the dome and around the edge, before being slipped into place.

When consistently used and properly fitted, conforming to the size and shape of your pelvis and your vaginal tissues, the diaphragm is about 85 to 95 per cent effective. But this figure remains hard to pin down because of possible human error (improper fit, insufficient foam or jelly, failure to leave in place long enough after intercourse, etc.)

As one woman reports, "I gained over 20 pounds last year after giving birth to my second child, but I didn't have my diaphragm refitted! And now my doctor tells me I'm pregnant again!" Moral: Any major weight gain or loss should bring you to your doctor for a refitting; the same applies after giving birth or having an abortion. Have your physician recheck your diaphragm once a year and inspect it periodically yourself—for any pin-sized holes or other signs of wear and tear. Rubber is subject to deterioration and requires care—after use it should be carefully washed, dried and put back in its covered case.

For the diaphragm to work, you must remember to apply fresh spermicide with an applicator for every act of intercourse and then leave the device in place for at least six hours afterward. Instead of allowing it to interfere, many couples have successfully integrated the diaphragm into their foreplay, enhancing pleasure for them both and making contraception a shared experience.

To decide whether a diaphragm is best for you, consider whether you're motivated to spend the time inserting, removing and maintaining it, or whether you are squeamish about touching yourself or slipping a device into your vagina. If you have persistent vaginitis or cystitis or an unusually shaped vagina, you may prefer another method.

Unlike the Pill or IUD, the diaphragm carries a very low risk of side effects because it does not alter the body chemically in any way. Women who use the diaphragm do have an increased likelihood of cystitis (bladder infections) and on rare occasions, users may be allergic to a spermicidal foam or cream or the rubber material.

The Condom

The principle here is a very simple and apparently time-honored one since Egyptians used some variation of the modern-day condom over 3,000 years ago. Italian scientist Giovanni Fallopio, for whom our Fallopian tubes have been named, is credited with having invented the first "official" condom back in 1500, though his purpose was to prevent venereal disease, not conception. (Sure enough, this contraceptive can help do both.)

Made of thin rubber latex or animal membrane, this sheath is slipped over an erect penis and worn during intercourse to prevent sperm from entering the vagina. Like the diaphragm, when used with a spermicidal jelly, it is highly effective.

As for drawbacks: Some couples complain that covering the penis with even the thinnest membrane diminishes sensation. Others find it awkward and disruptive, although as with the diaphragm, many couples incorporate the ritual into their lovemaking. Condoms sometimes break under the pressure of ejaculation so seminal fluid may escape. (Leaving extra room at the tip can help prevent this.)

A fresh condom should be used with every act of intercourse. Since semen may leak out almost any time, even before ejaculation occurs, the condom should be slipped on before the penis approaches the vagina. After ejaculation, a man must withdraw his penis quickly to prevent semen from spilling into or around the vagina.

For teenagers, apparently, the advantages outweigh the inconvenience: This is currently the most popular form of contraception among the 14- to 19-year-old age group, a rather welcome statistic, considering that this barrier method offers almost full protection against sexually transmitted disease. Twenty-five percent of all condom purchases are made by women.

Spermicidal Jelly, Cream, Foam, Suppositories

Inserted into the vagina, these contraceptives ward off pregnancy by throwing up a barricade of sperm-killing ingredients. Easy to apply, inexpensive and available over-the-counter, this is a popular category of contraceptives. Some complaints are of possible messiness or inconvenience since a fresh supply of each is needed for every act of intercourse.

One recent study has suggested a slightly increased risk of defective children born to women using spermicides at or several weeks before the time of conception. Allergy to the spermicides is also possible in a small percentage of users. When combined with the condom these chemical barriers provide excellent birth control.

The Vaginal Sponge

A more convenient takeoff on the familiar diaphragm, the disposable vaginal sponge is the newest addition to the arsenal of barrier contraceptives. Recently granted FDA approval and marketed under the trade name *Today*, it resembles a plumped-up powder puff and can be worn up to 24 hours before intercourse, thus allowing for unplanned encounters!

The sponge prevents pregnancy three ways: by blocking the cervix, killing the sperm and absorbing the ejaculate. Because it is already saturated with a spermicide, there is no need to apply cream or jelly, nor is reinsertion necessary with every act of sex. It is more compact, flexible and easier to insert than the diaphragm, and no "waiting period" is required. (Like the diaphragm it must be left in at least six hours before removal.)

Fitting by a physician is unnecessary, as one size—two inches in diameter—fits all. As for effectiveness, the sponge is roughly equivalent to the diaphragm if properly and consistently used; the failure rate with both devices is highest during the earliest months, so supplementary protection such as the condom is advised at the beginning. While the sponge comes with complete package instructions, women who have never used a vaginal contraceptive should see a family planning counselor or doctor for additional guidance.

Note: Since the sponge can be left in for a considerable length of time, some physicians have questioned its potential for causing toxic shock. (See Chapter 6.) However, laboratory tests so far show no evidence that the sponge promotes the growth of the bacterium (staph aureus) responsible for the disease. In addition, the spermicide used is antibacterial and its acidic makeup, similar to that of the vagina, should discourage the growth of the toxic-shock-related organism. (It may also inhibit the bacteria associated with venereal disease.) More thorough clinical testing will be conducted to evaluate this risk.

The Rhythm Method

As you have seen, ovulation marks a woman's fertile period—an "unsafe" interval if you are having sex and seeking to avoid pregnancy. If you are relying on the natural or "rhythm" method of birth control, you are required to monitor your monthly cycles continually to determine when to abstain from intercourse.

There are three ways to do this: by charting your basal body temperature (BBT) to pinpoint the time of ovulation (it drops just before an egg is released and rises noticeably shortly afterward); by checking your cervical mucus for telltale changes in texture that signal ovulation and/or by noting the length of your cycles and using a numerical formula to specify your fertile time (called simply the Calendar Method).

For this method to work, you should be well-motivated and willing to keep a careful record of bodily changes

135

throughout your cycle; obviously, you and your partner must also be willing to forego intercourse for a given time each month. Many couples explore other "creative" forms of lovemaking during this interval which actually enhance and broaden their sexual scenario.

Women whose periods are unpredictable and those coping with physical or emotional upsets or illness which could disrupt their menstrual regularity are not ideal candidates for the natural approach.

Drawbacks: While menstruation is unmistakable, ovulation does not necessarily give any direct, clear-cut sign. In a quarter of women, periods are frequently erratic and most women are irregular for some time after giving birth, so they are not well-suited for this method. Sometimes ovulation itself can result from the stimulus of sexual intercourse. Also, since sperm can survive in a woman's cervix for up to 72 hours and possibly even longer after sex, pregnancy can possibly result if intercourse occurs several days before ovulation. That's why relying on calendar dates alone is chancy at best. Combined with the temperature method, however, it can be very protective, with a success rate of up to 94 percent. By the time you record a temperature rise, the fertilization interval is usually over, indicating a relatively safe period until the next menstruation.

If you menstruated with perfect regularity, every 28 days, ovulation would most likely take place at the midpoint of the cycle, around the 14th day, but could occur anywhere from the 12th to the 17th—a six-day stretch. Because sperm may linger roughly 72 hours within a woman's body, about three days before this would also be an inadvisable time for intercourse. Add to this a full 24 hours *after* ovulation in which the sperm/egg rendezvous is still possible and you have a total of 6 plus 3 plus 1 = 10 days (from about the ninth to the 18th day of the cycle inclusive) during which you should abstain from sex.

The Cervical Cap

This small plastic or rubber device is designed to prevent conception by blocking the opening to the womb—a barrier method already practiced by European women for a number of years. Now, new tailor-made, precisely-sized variations of the European model, doctor-fitted from impressions made of a woman's cervix and equipped with a one-way valve to permit release of menstrual fluid, are being developed in this country. The innovations may allow the cap to remain in place for up to a full year, thereafter requiring annual "renewals" to maintain protection.

Working on a similar principle as the contact lens (which is held in place by the surface tension of occular fluid), the cap is supported by the suction of cervical fluid. As with the IUD, the cap will feature a marker so a woman can tell it's properly placed by checking from time to time.

Contraceptive Vaginal Ring

From developers at the Population Council, time-released, synthetic progestin via a small, flexible plastic ring, about two inches in diameter, can inhibit ovulation, fertilization and the implantation of an egg. It is designed to be self-inserted, high in the vagina near the cervix, reinserted after each period and reused for up to two years. Clinical trials of the ring are now being conducted in the U.S. and elsewhere.

Contraception According to Age

Even more than attitudes and personal preferences, age is a crucial variable in determining the most appropriate contraceptive. For example, many doctors do not want to insert an IUD in a woman who has not yet borne a child because of the heightened risk of ectopic pregnancy, and pelvic infection or inflammatory disease which could impair fertility. Because a good deal of teenage sex is sporadic and unplanned, the condom plus foam, readily available, easy to use, quite effective and protective against venereal disease, is probably the most suitable method for the under-20 age group. (This alternative also requires a man to become involved and take some responsibility for birth control.)

Actually, the Pill is least hazardous for women in their 20s and younger, although this is the group among whom decline in oral contraceptive use has been most notable in the wake of adverse publicity.

The second most popular strategy among younger couples is withdrawal before ejaculation, an unfortunate fact considering this method's notorious failure rate. While an increasing number of sexually active teens are resorting to birth control, their use of protection is still erratic and occasional. According to statistics compiled by the Alan Guttmacher Institute, only one third in this category have reported using contraception for *each* act of intercourse— either because the sexual episode was unexpected or because they simply thought pregnancy would not result from ''that one time.'' Some of the female respondents said they did not believe they were in the fertile part of their cycles when sex took place.

Before menopause, during the waning years of the menstrual cycle, oral contraceptives are rarely prescribed because their risks are considerable for this age group. Natural family planning is not advised either because there is no way of determining a completely ''safe'' interval during the premenopause when periods are irregular and unpredictable. The menopause itself is not defined as having taken place until a full year has elapsed since the last episode of menstrual bleeding. So, middle-aged, sexually active women must continue to use some form of contraception until they are *postmenopausal* (a condition best determined by your doctor).

Tubal ligation, today a vastly improved and simplified procedure which is even potentially reversible, may be appropriate for a woman in her late 30s or early 40s who has completed her family and firmly decided against future pregnancies. (Vasectomy for men, however, is an even safer, less complicated procedure.) The IUD is an acceptable alternative if surgery is not desired, though the device should not be left in place after the menopause. Barrier methods—condom, foam, diaphragm, sponge—are very effective during the premenopausal years when fertility is on the decline. After one year without menstruation, a woman may discontinue contraception altogether. (See also the chapter on menopause.)

When deciding on appropriate contraception at any age, it's important to be honest with yourself. "I knew I would have trouble with the Pill because I am notoriously absentminded," one of my patients confessed. "Sure enough, I forgot to take it on two consecutive days—with disastrous results! I became pregnant and had to have an abortion. Other times, I've been plagued with breakthrough bleeding because I've missed a Pill here and there. I also have a very hectic schedule which doesn't help, either!"

It took an unwanted pregnancy to make her establish a strict daily routine that would prevent any such accidents thereafter! Consider whether your lifestyle, temperament, idiosyncrasies and the like will permit you to adopt a given birth control method with a minimum of mishap.

ON THE MEDICAL HORIZON: CONTRACEPTION BREAKTHROUGHS

Ongoing research is yielding new refinements all the time in the science of contraception—the making of more reliable, convenient, comfortable, safer and longer-lasting methods to suit a wide range of needs and preferences. Many current research efforts are at various stages of development— being tested in a laboratory, undergoing clinical trials both here and overseas or still on the medical drawing board. Here is an update on the imminent and more distant breakthroughs.

Contraception by Injection or Implant

Both the U.S. and several foreign countries are testing a time-released, birth control drug which slowly emits a synthetic progesterone (progestin) to offer protection for at least six months. The compound, Norethindrone, is administered in the form of tiny pellets implanted under the skin of the forearm (an easy in-office technique) or by injection of microscopic quantities of hormones.

Norethindrone prevents pregnancy by halting ovulation or altering the hormone sequence that regulates menstruation. The drug is also believed to act on the lining of the uterus to prevent a fertilized egg from taking root. The implant or injection poses relatively few known risks to health (it bypasses the gastrointestinal tract and thus may minimize side effects). However, women who are strictly prohibited from using the Pill may not be candidates for this method, either.

At the end of six months' usage, the effects of the drug wear off from the body, presumably permitting future fertility (unless a woman is reinjected). It may take a certain length of time to conceive after discontinuing, as the chemicals must clear the bloodstream completely first.

Researchers are expected to have final test results within one year in order to meet FDA standards. Within the next decade, scientists intend to develop safer, smaller implants consisting of easily eliminated, biodegradable materials, that would provide continual protection for five to 10 years. Such a drug is reportedly being tested now in Mexico with no documented side effects.

Also on the horizon are anti-pregnancy vaccines designed for six to twelve months' protection, followed up by periodic "boosters." The principle at work is to spur the body's own immune system to develop antibodies against sperm, eggs or the hormones needed to sustain a pregnancy. For example, HCG is produced by the placenta and picks up where progesterone leaves off, to maintain a growing fetus starting from several weeks after conception to the end of pregnancy.

On women tested so far, the anti-HCG shot does not result in perceptible side effects, though some subjects simply don't respond to the vaccine. Others do have the expected immunological reaction, manufacturing their own "anti-pregnancy" hormones soon after being injected.

Prostaglandins and Birth Control

Can prostaglandins provide a foolproof answer to birth control? So far, the evidence has been encouraging enough to result in the establishment of a World Health Organization–sponsored committee to investigate the possibility. What we do know already: For women who have had intercourse without contraceptive protection, prostaglandins administered a few days after the first missed period are reported to trigger normal periodic bleeding within a few hours.

Present in the amniotic fluid surrounding the fetus, certain prostaglandins (similar to those that give rise to monthly cramps) cause strong muscular and uterine contractions which induce labor. They have been the basis of drugs used for this purpose (on a limited basis) in the U.S. and in Great Britain for both full-term births and therapeutic abortions during the second trimester.

Several years ago, Dr. Josef Fried of the University of Chicago announced that he had successfully synthesized a safe and completely effective prostaglandin contraceptive called the F2 Alpha analog (a variant of the natural F2 Alpha prostaglandin normally found in the body). A woman would need to take this pill only once a month and many researchers predict that, unlike existing morning after or even regular Pills, this one would produce no serious problems.

The prostaglandin pill recently tested by Dr. Fried and Dr. John McCracken of the Worcester Foundation of Experimental Biology in Shrewsbury, Massachusetts. (where the first birth control pill was developed in 1956) causes no muscle contractions as do the abortion-inducing prostaglandins. Instead, it depresses the ovaries' progesterone production. (Without progesterone, a natural hormone which fluctuates during a woman's cycle, it is difficult for a fertilized egg to implant in the uterus.)

The F2 Alpha pill can be taken to prevent a pregnancy or to terminate an existing one since, whether or not conception has already taken place, it will have the same effect of artificially reducing the body's progesterone level and bringing on the menstrual flow. (This pill would not terminate pregnancy after roughly the fifth or sixth week of gestation, when the placenta starts to manufacture its own progesterone.) When menstruation is precipitated by the drug *after* conception has taken place, an embryo in the uterus will simply be passed from the body. At such an early stage of development (at most about two to three weeks), it would be an imperceptible group of cells, but some anti-abortionists may well find this objectionable. In any case, when a prostaglandin birth-control pill is approved and marketed, it could become the safest, most convenient and reliable method available—and just as quickly the focus of an enormous controversy.

Contraceptive Tampons?

A tampon-like device saturated with a spermicide and wearable up to several days before intercourse is being studied by Excelsior Laboratories in New York City. Since the sperm-killing agent is released only during sexual contact, potential for irritation is minimal. The ejaculate is also absorbed rather swiftly by the tampon—within minutes after intercourse. Clinical trials both here and abroad have so far been very promising.

Peptides: The Nasal
Spray Contraceptive

As you have seen, the whole menstrual cycle begins with the hypothalamus. This undistinguished-looking portion of the brain, situated right above the pituitary gland, sends out small proteins or peptides known as "releasing factors" that awaken the pituitary to secrete its own sex-gland-arousing hormones, FSH and LH. As a result, the egg-producing ovaries are stimulated to produce estrogen and progesterone. The very same sequence works for men; the difference being that FSH and LH are summoned to activate the testes or storehouse for sperm.

Having traced the pathway leading to conception, scientists are now working on a way to prevent fertility through some chemical manipulation. To this end, they have developed synthetic peptides which, at certain dosages, can prod the pituitary just like the natural kinds. However, given in large amounts, they have a paradoxical effect: fooling the pituitary into thinking that the level of FSH and LH in the body is excessive, thereby influencing it to secrete *less* of these two chemicals. As a result, both sperm and egg production are inhibited.

These peptides, in the form of a daily nasal spray, have been studied in Sweden as a contraceptive for both women and men. Fertility should return when the spraying stops, generally by the time of the next one or two menstrual periods in women and after a roughly equivalent interval in men.

Different forms of the peptides—injectable, intervaginal and under the tongue—will be tested here and the National

Institutes Of Health has funded two research programs in the U.S. to determine these synthetic chemicals' safety and reliability after long-term use.

New Forms of the Pill and the IUD

Physicians now acknowledge that synthetic estrogens may be to blame for many side effects currently associated with the Pill, so research is now investigating the use of natural estrogens instead (similar to those in hormone replacement therapy). Also being developed are a number of "multiphase" pills that more closely conform to natural hormonal ups and downs throughout the month and which may minimize such problems as breakthrough bleeding. In addition, a number of non-estrogen compounds—designed to be taken at the end of a given menstrual cycle and to inhibit ovulation or prevent fertilization or implantation— are being explored as possible once-a-month Pills. For example, as noted above, the F2 Alpha analog, which thwarts implantation by inducing a kind of "labor," is intended for one-time use every month.

IUDs soaked with progestins may allow them to remain effective and intact for longer than the two-to-three year current limit; the progesterone itself may also help eliminate the common side effect of heavy menstrual bleeding and cramping.

SANS CONTRACEPTION

Just what are the chances of becoming pregnant if you have used no birth control at all during mid-cycle or your so-called fertile period? This all depends on the fertility potential of you *and* your partner, not just you alone, according to Robert A. Wild, M.D., assistant professor, department of obstretrics and gynecology at the University of Tennessee College of Medicine in Knoxville, (as recently reported in *Medical Aspects of Human Sexuality*).

An estimated 50 percent of fertility problems are believed to originate with men; and 30 to 50 percent of the time, a combination dysfunction may be at fault. However, assuming that both of you have a problem-free potential for childbearing, your chances of conceiving are 25 percent if you have intercourse every other day. Two thirds of normally functioning women are expected to conceive within six months at this rate. Obviously, the more often intercourse takes place, the greater your odds of becoming pregnant.

Chapter 8

DIET AND THE MENSTRUAL CYCLE

One basic definitely bears repeating: The better your diet, the greater your energy, stamina, well-being and capacity to resist or overcome any bodily complaints—including those related to your monthly cycle. Along with a chronically stressful lifestyle, poor eating habits may contribute to menstrual distress—so keeping your nutritional house in order is essential to healthy menstruation.

It has been reported that premenstrual syndrome, painful cramps and menopausal problems are less common in vegetarian societies, and that women who alter their diets by cutting back on meats often claim their condition improves. No one can yet explain why this might be so, but perhaps certain foods or eating patterns are responsible for elevating undesirable prostaglandins or suppressing the release of benevolent ones, or for balancing lopsided hormones. At this point, scientists do not know whether diet, genetic makeup or some other unsuspected factor(s) can account for why some women with primary dysmenorrhea or PMS show abnormal prostaglandin and/or hormone levels compared to women without symptoms. But if manipulating a diet can help change body chemistry and alleviate or aggravate certain symptoms, then maybe it *is* a major link in the chain of menstrual events. (At least one nutrient/chemical connection has been established: progesterone synthesis is dependent on vitamin A, among other ingredients.)

As reported in the chapter on premenstrual syndrome, the most advisable eating strategy during the premenstrual week involves frequent smaller meals consisting of high protein and complex carbohydrates, with no refined sugars or starches and a minimum of salt and exotic spices. For protein, good alternatives to red meats include grains, seafood, poultry, low-fat dairy products (also excellent for calcium) and legumes (in moderation). Another source, desiccated liver, has the advantage of being cholesterol-free.

If bloating is a special problem, indulge in the naturally diuretic foods such as asparagus, watercress, cucumber, parsley, artichoke, eggplant, watermelon and cranberry juice, along with a generous amount of filtered water or seltzer (sodium-free). While it sounds paradoxical, water is probably the very best diuretic of all. Ample potassium, available in fresh oranges and ripe bananas, (and such foods as the white meat of chicken, tomato juice, dried fruits; lentils and raw carrots) will also counterbalance sodium and curb the body's tendency to hold back water during this time. Dr. Barbara Edelstein, author of *The Woman Doctor's Diet Book for Women*, recommends one carbohydrate-free day for particularly stubborn fluid retention, "to help flush out the system."

Besides excess water, constipation can intensify both cramping and premenstrual discomfort, so make sure your diet includes foods that will help keep bowels loose—prunes, apricots, apples, figs, a small amount of wheat bran (too much of the latter may irritate the gastrointestinal tract and interfere with calcium absorption if dairy foods are eaten at the same time.) Dieters should bear in mind that dried fruits, though effective laxatives, are relatively high in calories; fresh fruits and raw vegetables, staples in any sensible, healthful diet, should provide enough natural roughage anyway, especially if you are not clogging your system with pasty white starches and sugars.

During your period, particularly if your flow is heavy or frequent, you may want to ensure against possible loss of iron with such wholesome choices as eggs, milk, apricots, peaches, prunes, organ meats (sparingly here), oysters, clams, kidney beans, kelp (in fresh or tablet form) and soybeans. If none of these foods are palatable, take a supplement such as FemIron or Stresstabs 600. (Iron is most efficiently absorbed by the body in the presence of vitamin C and/or E.) A light diet featuring freshly squeezed vegetable and fruit juices and low-fat dairy foods may be easiest on the digestive tract during the first few days of menstruation.

Calcium is one of the most frequently recommended supplements for both cramps and premenstrual distress, as well as for the premenopausal years (and after) when estrogen is on the wane. Calcium is one of the body's macrominerals, required in generous amounts for a variety of crucial functions, among them, contractions of muscle tissue, the transmission of nerve impulses and the regulation of blood pressure. Calcium is reported to be at its lowest about 10 days before the period begins, so the need for supplements and foods rich in the mineral seems to be greatest at this time. Outright calcium deficiency has been linked with leg and uterine cramps, water retention, irritability, nervous tension and headaches. Sure enough, restoring calcium has been associated with the relief of these and other annoying symptoms. Calcium-rich foods include dairy products, seafood and leafy greens.

In the body, calcium functions best in a roughly two-to-one ratio with its complementary mineral magnesium. So if you are taking supplements, try to keep your intake within the same proportions. As mentioned in Chapter 4, certain foods interfere with calcium absorption such as spinach, which contains the mineral-binding oxalic acid, along with excess wheat fiber, protein and phosphorus.

GTF-chromium, a supplement which helps stabilize blood sugar, has been used to treat women with hard-to-control premenstrual cravings and the fatigue, irritability, palpitations and headache associated with temporary disturbances in fuel metabolism.

Zinc and selenium, both considered important minerals

at menopause, function as *antioxidants:* substances which counteract the cell-damaging, decay-promoting effects of oxygen within the body. Scientists now suspect that including adequate amounts of such nutrients in the daily diet over a number of years may help retard the cellular aging process, a theory already bolstered by a number of controlled animal experiments. They may even curb the development of degenerative illnesses such as cancer and heart disease. Zinc is supplied by milk, shellfish, oats, lamb, string beans, lettuce, cucumbers, beans, potatoes, tuna and many nuts. Selenium is supplied by shellfish, wheat germ and bran, barley, citrus fruits, mushrooms, onions, kidney beans, green beans, radishes and cottage cheese.

Other important antioxidants (which reinforce each other's effects) are vitamin C, E, members of the B-complex such as B1, B5 and B6 and vitamin A. Vitamin C is crucial to strong, elastic blood vessel walls and healthy cell membranes—important to a well-functioning reproductive system. In foods, other factors usually occur together with vitamin C—particularly bioflavinoids, rutin and hesperidin. These elements (sometimes called P factors or parts of the "C complex") are blood-vessel strengtheners that may be helpful to women who bleed copiously during menstruation (a condition called menorrhagia). Food sources include green peppers and the white pulpy part of citrus fruits; a number of·supplements feature C and these complementary factors together.

Even more common than iron loss during the childbearing years is a relative shortage of folic acid (a member of the B complex), reports Dr. Richard A. Kunin, author of *Mega-Nutrition for Women* (McGraw-Hill), especially for women on the Pill. The versatile vitamin B6 is likewise depleted by oral contraceptives, along with smoking and alcohol. As already noted in the chapter on PMS, B6 is often given to ease nausea and premenstrual fluid buildup (particularly swelling of the breast and abdomen) and to help maintain blood sugar on an even keel. In some cases, B6 has been reported effective against menstruation-related acne. Strict vegetarians who eschew cheese and eggs must supplement their diets with vitamin B12 since it can only be obtained in foods from animal sources.

Vitamin E, a fat-soluble nutrient, is a preserver of the fatty portions of the cell, complementing the antioxidant properties of water-soluble vitamin C and the B-complex. It is also essential to a healthy circulatory system. Most recently, it has been found effective against fibrocystic lumps of the breast which are most uncomfortable during the premenstrual phase.

ON SUPPLEMENTS

For women with busy schedules, job-related stresses and demanding family obligations, planning meals with care to provide all necessary nutrients may be impractical, if not impossible. A recent survey by the U.S. Department of Agriculture found that it simply isn't possible for a woman to meet even the minimal requirements represented by the RDA levels of vitamins and minerals if she is consuming less than 1,600 calories a day. So many of us are perennially dieting and mindful of calories that we aren't coming anywhere near this figure. If you *are* watching your weight, supplements are necessary to ensure adequate intake of all nutrients. Obesity and consumption of more than 1,600 calories does not necessarily mean that you are eating sensibly, of course. Overindulgence in sweets or fatty foods can result in imbalances and shortages of key vitamins and minerals in the long run.

Oral contraceptives, alcohol, smoking, stress, medications, infections, menstrual blood losses and chronic illnesses, among other influences, may elevate the body's requirement for certain nutrients. Also, most of us rely heavily on convenience foods—packaged, canned, frozen, processed— as well as the produce from the local supermarket which is often shipped considerable distances and/or held in storage for a length of time before arriving on grocery shelves.

Not surprisingly, the nutrient content of such foods is often substantially reduced by the time we eat them. In other cases, convenience foods are "fortified" with a few key vitamins and minerals in an attempt to restore what has been depleted—but too often the enzymes, micronutrients, trace elements, fiber and other factors are not included.

Even if a diet were consistently to provide the RDAs of all the nutrients (originally designed for some mythical normal individual), a growing number of physicians, biochemists and nutrition professionals are questioning whether these basic levels are really sufficient to ensure optimum health, and not merely defensive protection against deficiency diseases. Finally, recent revelations about nutrition's role in the etiology of such serious conditions as cancer of the colon and the breast and cardiovascular disease should also cause more physicians and patients alike to consider diet a very important, controllable and too-often overlooked contributor to lifelong health and well-being.

WEIGHT LOSS AND THE MENSTRUAL CYCLE

As any dieter and her physician know, certain times of the menstrual cycle can interfere with serious efforts to lose weight. Any calorie-conserving eating plan for menstruating women should take into account the cyclical metabolic changes and shifting hormone ratios that can have an impact on the way the body handles fats, fluids and calories, or on its levels of energy, appetite or mood.

During the week or so before menstruation, cravings for sweet or salty foods, moodiness, depression and/or accelerated water retention can sabotage even the most dedicated dieter. You may reach a maddening plateau just when you are trying your hardest—after days of steady weight loss your scale refuses to budge or even shows a marked increase because of water-logged tissues! Or you may have a sudden, uncontrollable urge to binge after having towed the line for so long.

As Dr. Edelstein points out, premenstrual water retention is related to fluctuating hormone levels and not simply to food and fluid intake. It can account for a gain of as much as four to five pounds, just when you are striving to cut back on calories. Even worse, the more water a woman conserves, the less fat she seems to lose, says Dr. Edelstein. "During her periods of greater water retention, her whole fat-burning system slows down and may virtually stop." Mainly for this reason, "You are five times more likely to go off a diet before your period than at any other time in your cycle," she adds.

Estrogen, refined carbohydrates, salt, alcohol and certain drugs, including the Pill, cortisone and antibiotics, will aid and abet this fluid-holding process. Oral contraceptives also make it easier for your body to convert food into fat, Dr. Edelstein claims: If you have been maintaining your weight on 1,600 calories a day, for example, and you start taking the Pill, you may have to cut your daily intake by about 160 calories (a reduction of 10 per cent) just to stay at the same level. Added to the normal "rebound" phenomenon that occurs after the first week on almost any diet, the results can be downright discouraging.

Dieting itself and any attempt to alter your eating patterns can affect the timing of your cycle. If you were previously regular, losing weight could make you temporarily irregular or vice versa; you may also ovulate sooner or later as a result, thus rendering any tried-and-true "rhythm" method of birth control suddenly less reliable!

How best to handle the frustrating premenstrual interval? Follow the eating guidelines suggested on p. 154 to keep fluid retention, cravings and other saboteurs to a minimum and observe a sensible weight-loss diet such as the one shown on pp. 156–161 with your physician's permission or that of a qualified nutrition professional. (Have a complete medical checkup before embarking on any weight-reducing regimen.)

The way to stabilize and maintain blood sugar is not by resorting to sugar itself: This will send your glucose level up, but the effect is short-lived, and it soon plummets to a point even lower than before.

When you hit a plateau, consistent aerobic exercise seems to make all the difference: It will help you alter your metabolic clock, eventually "resetting" it at a faster rate so you can lose pounds more efficiently.

It's also wise to lower your expectations during your premenstrual phase and to acknowledge this interval as a temporary slowdown or stopping point, as a time when you're more susceptible to dietary setbacks, through no fault of your own but rather as a result of natural bodily changes. If you allow for this biological reality, rather than trying to resist it and becoming discouraged, you will probably get through the interval with your emotional equilibrium—and resolve—intact. Realize that if you simply persevere, and are extra-vigilant at this time, weight loss will eventually proceed as it did before.

The good news: Your body's water weight and appetite level are at their *lowest* when menstruation begins.

SOME DIET GUIDELINES

Whenever possible, plan meals to include a wide variety of foods and with an eye to conserving nutrients. That means eating raw, unpeeled fruits and vegetables, using them in blended drinks or else cooking minimally—steaming, stir-frying or boiling for short periods in small amounts of water. (Save the cooking water for soups and stews.) Do not store fresh produce or fruit juices for more than a few days in the refrigerator, as they lose vitamins rapidly. Buy them in small quantities so you will use them up right away and not forget you have them.

Remember, the best natural diuretic is water, straight from the tap (with a filter attached to screen out harmful additives) or a bottled kind such as seltzer (triple-filtered and sodium-free), Volvic or Poland Springs. About four glasses a day should help keep your water-excreting systems flowing smoothly! Beware of diet sodas while you are premenstrual or losing weight; they are relatively high in sodium, the leading villain in fluid retention.*

As you have seen in the chapter on menstrual irregularities, both too much and too little body weight can be undesirable for your reproductive system. Chronic underweight and stringent dieting can even halt your periods altogether (amenorrhea) or result in scanty, infrequent bleeding (oligomenorrhea). This temporary shutdown is believed to be a protective mechanism which prevents conception when the body is inadequately equipped to support and nourish a fetus. Both conditions are reversible if enough weight is regained.

As for appearance's sake, a loss of too much body fat causes thinning of the skin's subcutaneous layer (beneath the dermis and epidermis), making the skin look less smooth and elastic; your facial contours gaunt and prematurely aged.

For help in losing weight safety, slowly and efficiently, you might follow the diet menu plan featured here below, with your physician's permission, of course.

Regardless of your weight-loss goals, avoid skipping meals. Eating three times a day (with healthful, low-calorie snacking in between if you are premenstrual) is essential to the success of any diet. For example, studies have shown that people who miss breakfast actually have a harder time losing weight because their body tries to over-compensate for the lost meal by retaining calories more efficiently, or else their hunger pangs induce them to overeat at the very next meal.

If you thrive best on six small meals a day, especially during the week before menstruation, divide your portions,

---

*Other healthful beverage choices include decaffeinated coffee or tea, herb tea, fresh fruit or vegetable juice and skim milk. (The latter is already indicated on the menu plan.)

eating part and saving the rest for about two hours later. Or, without adding too many additional calories, follow the three-meal format featured here and choose such wholesome snacks as the following to handle cravings. These might include plain chilled yogurt with mixed fresh fruits (delicious!); cold unsweetened cereal with skim milk; carrot sticks or apple slices flavored with cinammon; a small bran muffin; a 2-oz. wedge of part-skim milk cheese (such as feta or Jarlsberg) on whole-wheat crackers; celery filled with low-fat cottage cheese and chopped scallions; or a thin slice of turkey or cheese wrapped around your favorite vegetable. With a little imagination, you can come up with many more palate-pleasing combinations.

Whenever you're dieting, if you find you're losing weight at too fast a pace or wish to maintain your current weight, add a few more grains, "snacks", fruits and/or starchy vegetables to your eating plan or increase entree portions slightly at lunch and dinner. If you are not losing weight, try cutting back your calorie intake by about 250 calories, which should add up to a loss of about ½ pound over a 7-day period. You should *always* be under the supervision of a physician or a well-qualified nutritionist if you are staying on *any* reducing plan for longer than seven days.

THE HEALTHY MENSTRUATING WOMAN'S DIET

Monday

Breakfast

½ fresh grapefruit
⅔ cup oatmeal with ½ cup skim milk, cinnamon and 1 small sliced banana or ¼ cup blueberries or an equivalent serving of any other fresh fruit of your choice plus 1 tablespoon toasted wheat germ or bran.

Lunch

4 ozs. curried chicken or tuna salad (4 ozs. cooked, diced skinless chicken or white meat tuna) with 1 tablespoon of plain yogurt, 1 teaspoon curry powder, ¼ cup fresh or drained canned pineapple, chopped celery and onion, apple chunks, a few raisins and bits of shredded coconut. Blend together well and serve over a bed of alfalfa sprouts, spinach or Romaine leaves.

1 small pita bread round (optional)
½ cup skim milk

Dinner

¼ roasted chicken basted with small amount of white wine, olive oil and fresh herbs
½ cup each steamed zucchini, Chinese cabbage
Artichoke hearts and pimiento salad
For "dessert" (optional) a small dish of dried fruits— apricots, prunes, dates or figs.

Tuesday

Breakfast

½ cup fresh strawberries or 1 medium orange with ½ cup plain yogurt.
1 egg prepared in non-stick pan (any style) with herbs for flavoring
1 small slice sprouted wheat bread

Lunch

Salad of assorted fresh vegetables (red cabbage, sprouts, tomatoes, cucumbers, green peppers, carrots, etc.) garnished with slices of fresh fruit, then topped with 3 ounces farmer or low-fat cottage cheese. To "dress up" vegetables, use yogurt, lemon juice, fresh dill and other herbs or add 1 tablespoon bottled low-calorie dressing of your choice.

Dinner

4 oz. baked flounder filet
½ cup each steamed broccoli and cauliflower with 1 teaspoon soft sweet butter or margarine
½ cup red potato salad with chopped fresh herbs, dash olive oil
1 fresh apple or pear

Wednesday

Breakfast

1 slice whole-wheat French toast
½ cantaloupe

½ cup skim milk

Lunch

4 ozs. sliced fresh turkey, thin slice Swiss cheese and shredded lettuce or sprouts with 1 slice pita or protein bread (made without shortening)
½ cup cucumber and tomato salad with sliced onions
½ cup fresh fruit salad

Dinner

4 ozs. pasta with tomato sauce, prepared with 1 tablespoon olive oil, fresh basil and garlic, topped with 1 oz. freshly grated Parmesan cheese
½ cup each steamed carrots and zucchini
Small tossed salad with watercress, celery and red pepper, lemon juice dressing
Small bunch grapes

Thursday

Breakfast

1 slice rye toast with ¼ cup cottage cheese, sprinkled with cinnamon
½ cup sliced fresh apricots
½ cup skim milk

Lunch

1 cup bean soup
3 ozs. water-packed salmon tossed with pimiento slices, onion, celery, cucumber, fresh dill and plain yogurt over Romaine leaves or alfalfa sprouts
Melon wedge
½ cup skim milk

Dinner

4–6 ozs. broiled shoulder lamb chops
½ cup brown rice cooked in beef or chicken broth
½ cup assorted steamed vegetables, e.g., cauliflower, Brussels sprouts, green beans with 1 pat melted butter or margarine
½ cup mandarin orange sections

Friday

Breakfast

1 medium orange or grapefruit (or 1 cup fresh squeezed orange or grapefruit juice)
1 egg prepared any style in non-stick pan
1 slice whole-grain bread with (optional) 1 tsp. soft butter or margarine
½ cup skim milk

Lunch

1 medium chef's salad
Fresh pineapple slices or other fruit in season
½ cup skim milk

Dinner

½ baked cornish hen with orange slices
8 asparagus spears
1 medium baked potato with 1 tablespoon plain yogurt, chopped
fresh chives and parsley
½ cup fresh fruit salad

Saturday

Breakfast

1 medium tangerine
Milk "shake" (1 cup skim milk, 1 egg, vanilla, 2 tbsps. plain
yogurt, 1 tbsp. toasted wheat germ, (cinnamon and nutmeg,
blended with ice cubes, if desired). For variations, add any
fresh fruit of your choice
1 buckwheat pancake with 1 tsp. butter or margarine

Lunch

½ cup chicken salad on 1 slice whole-wheat toast
½ cup steamed yellow squash
½ cup skim milk

Dinner

4 ozs. steamed mussels with lemon juice
1 cup Romaine salad with 1 tablespoon garbanzo beans and
carrot slices
½ cup wild rice
1 medium peach
½ cup plain frozen yogurt with fresh strawberries

Sunday

Breakfast

1 medium orange
½ cup whole-grain cereal with raisins, dried fruit and skim milk
1 oz. Monterey Jack cheese

Lunch

1 cup fresh chopped vegetables with 1 sliced hard-cooked egg, turkey and cheese (chop 1 slice of each and add to salad) and 2 tablespoons bulghur wheat, lemon juice dressing
1 slice pumpernickel bread with 1 pat butter or margarine
½ cup fresh fruit salad
½ cup skim milk

Dinner

4 ozs. broiled veal chops
1 cup chickory salad with green beans
1 medium baked potato with dill
½ cup sliced, unpeeled apples with plain yogurt and granola topping

A ONCE-A-MONTH GUIDE TO
HEALTHY SKIN

Chapter 9

YOUR ONCE-A-MONTH GUIDE TO HEALTHY SKIN

One of the most obvious ways your monthly cycle manifests itself is through your body's outer envelope and largest organ—the skin. A mirror of internal functions, your skin shows changes in texture, tone and permeability as hormones fluctuate throughout the month. Oil glands may become more or less active with cyclical changes as well.

In the week or two before menstruation, you may notice that your skin breaks out easily—literally overnight—or is more prone to oiliness. These premenstrual acne flareups are experienced by roughly one half of those women already coping with facial pimples. (Remember, acne itself is not simply a disease of adolescence but may linger on well into prime-time adulthood or first flourish in the 20s, 30s or even later.) Although the number of pimples does not vary dramatically throughout a given month, the rhythm of their appearance and disappearance often follows a cyclical pattern.

While no one knows for sure, doctors believe that the premenstrual surge in progesterone, a hormone chemically similar to androgens or male hormones, is responsible for activating the oil or sebum-producing glands which can result in acne. Everyone's skin harbors thousands of tiny sebaceous glands at birth, particularly in the face, chest and back, but it is not until puberty that the sudden onrush of male hormones or androgens present in both sexes awakens and enlarges the dormant glands, reports Dr. Fredric Haberman, a leading New York dermatologist and co-author of *Your Skin: A Dermatologist's Guide to a Lifetime of Beauty and Health* (Berkley, 1983). Though the resulting flow of oil does not automatically lead to acne, it is the necessary "fuel" and no pimples are possible without it. Some newborn babies have shown chins full of acne because their bloodstream still bears traces of troublemaking maternal hormones. (This "cradle acne" generally clears up on its own within several weeks or months.)

While hormones play the role of instigator, usually no imbalance, excess or deficit of any kind is involved. Only a small amount is needed to promote the acne process and often it is impossible to distinguish the androgen levels of acne patients from those of clear-skinned types.

Both progesterone and circulating male hormones are converted by enzymes into a potent substance called *dihydrotestosterone,* the factor most directly responsible for stimulating the oil glands. So with more progesterone available in the two weeks before menstruation, acne is more likely to erupt during this interval than any other. (Scientists have speculated that someday, acne may be controlled or even prevented if we find a way to counteract the effects of dihydrotestosterone on the sebaceous glands without tampering with the body's hormone makeup.)

Just the opposite may hold for the first two weeks into the cycle, however, when estrogen predominates. Estrogen has an inhibiting effect on sebum production, which is why pregnant women and those on high-dose oral contraceptives often watch their acne disappear.

In fact, some doctors prescribe estrogen-dominant birth control pills for a limited period of time for women with severe acne who have failed to respond to more conventional therapy. (The hormone's effects are too "feminizing" to allow its use on men.) This is considered a last-resort treatment except for those women who elect contraception via the Pill, cautions Dr. Haberman. Also, a patient may not see significant improvement until the third or fourth month, and in fact may look worse at the very beginning (for reasons not clearly understood) before she gets better, he adds. If a woman is on the Pill already and then decides to seek treatment for acne, she should tell her dermatologist what kind of contraceptive formula she has been using. Often, just switching to a relatively high estrogen/low progestin pill goes a long way toward avoiding or clearing up the acne which would otherwise have occurred periodically.

A significant number of women are *not* helped by the Pill, regardless of how it's formulated, and there is no way of telling beforehand who will and who won't respond. And withdrawal from any kind of Pill may cause a sudden flareup due to a rebound reaction as the body adjusts to new hormone levels. The same phenomenon may occur after childbirth, with equally visible impact on the skin.

Since men obviously have more testosterone, their oil glands are larger and more active—and they are generally more prone to acne, including its severe, cystic forms. Also, sebum production falls off only slightly in men as they age, whereas it decreases dramatically in women after the age of 50.

Occasionally the onset of acne in adulthood can signal the presence of pituitary, adrenal or ovarian tumors. The condition will usually be accompanied by other signs of excess androgen or erratic hormone activity: irregular menstrual periods, the growth of facial hair, deepening of the voice and other anomalies.

How to cope with premenstrual breakouts? Wash your face with warm, soapy water and pat dry with a clean towel or tissues. Never rub pimples vigorously or attempt to pick or remove them yourself; otherwise you run the risk of irritating them further, and possibly causing them to rupture internally, incurring the risk of permanent scarring.

A simple cleansing ritual two to three times a day, followed by some dabbing with alcohol or store-bought benzoyl peroxide, a topical drying/mildly antibacterial agent, should be sufficient to keep these blemishes under control.

Be aware that some cosmetics will aggravate or instigate acne because they are formulated with irritating or oily, skin-clogging ingredients. (Ironically, many women use cosmetics and vanishing creams to cover up their acne, only to find that these trigger still more outbreaks, leading to a vicious cycle.) Your safest bet if you're prone to premenstrual pimples is to use water-based or oil-free foundations. You can usually recognize the former as liquids that separate when not in use and have to be shaken. Because oil-free (alcohol-based) makeups contain emulsifiers (which hold the ingredients together), they are less likely to cake or turn pasty than the water-based kinds. However, the emulsifiers that make them more cosmetically elegant aggravate existing acne in some people, warns Dr. Haberman. Try an oil-free foundation if you find it more appealing, he suggests, but study your face closely and switch brands if one product seems to provoke a skin eruption. Generally, makeups containing pigments, water, glycerine, alcohol and propylene glycol are best choices for acne-sensitive skin.

OTHER "FEMALE" SKIN PROBLEMS

Melasma, also called chloasna, gravidarum or the mask of pregnancy, is the term for mottled, liver-spotted skin, especially on the face, forehead and temples, that may be triggered by oral contraceptives, pregnancy or repeated sun exposure. These flat, smooth, brownish and entirely harmless blemishes (unlike moles, they can never turn malignant) are larger than freckles and up to several inches in diameter. While they often disappear spontaneously, complete clearing may take up to a year. If the condition is precipitated by pregnancy, it usually vanishes within a few months of delivery. However, melasma resulting from the Pill has been known to last up to five years after a woman has stopped using oral contraceptives.

Sunscreens will help prevent them and bleaching creams (preferably the prescription kind) containing hydroxyquinone help fade them away. They can also be removed with an electric needle or a mild acid peeling agent followed by a specially prepared bleaching formula. Patients must be warned, however, that post-inflammatory hyperpigmentation (further darkening) can result from some of these procedures.

Hormone-related skin changes may also include hair problems—too much or too little. During puberty, when glands are working overtime, a young girl's body sometimes becomes "confused" and produces excessive androgen. Girls with this disorder characteristically have erratic menstrual periods, underdeveloped breasts and too much facial hair. Your physician can usually determine whether adrenal or ovarian malfunction is the underlying cause. When the problem is successfully treated, the unwanted hair may fall out on its own with minimal hair growth or may require removal by electrolysis.

Abnormal thinning or loss of hair may be the result of too much androgen—and the imbalance seems to be on the rise in women, Dr. Haberman explains. "Some women inherit strong genes (for thinning hair) from one or both parents. You might say they are 'programmed' for this condition, and as years go by they may begin to lose some or a great deal of hair, especially from the sides and top of the scalp," he says. "Others may or may not have these troublesome genes but do not lose their hair unless or until something triggers an increase in male hormones in their bodies.

"That 'something' could be emotional stress," the doctor adds, "which raises the level of male hormones in women. In fact, the tense times we live in could well be responsible for the increase in female androgenic baldness. Other culprits can be found among the 140-odd pharmaceuticals that are also male-hormone stimulants." (Oddly, these same androgen-arousing drugs are also often a factor in acne and hirsutism, resulting in too much oil and hair on the face and body, where neither is welcomed, and too little on the scalp, of course.) While mostly associated with midlife, the hair-thinning syndrome can begin well before, sometimes even in the late 20s and early 30s.

Right now, scientists are investigating ways of counteracting the damage done by the bloodstream's free-wheeling androgens through various chemical strategies—mostly still on the medical drawing board. Meanwhile, dermatologists recommend stress reduction, the elimination of androgenic compounds, and for severe, widespread hair loss, transplants, may be an alternative. (Only a dermatologist can tell for sure whether someone is a good transplant candidate. His first job is to determine the type and cause of the patient's hair loss.)

Recently, a blood pressure lowering drug called Aldactone has been found to curb the activity of the hair-thinning androgens, an unexpected side effect. Another hypertension-fighting drug, Minoxidil, may promote hair growth in some patients who receive standard therapeutic doses. It is currently being tested in clinical trials as a treatment for baldness, and results so far are inconclusive.

CAN HORMONES MAKE YOU LOOK YOUNGER?

Some women have sought treatment with hormone replacement therapy (see Chapter 5) because they believe that "estrogen will make my skin look younger." Well, it's not that simple and no one knows for certain. The most we can say, given present knowledge, is that hormone replacements will most likely not hurt your skin and may help you partially preserve the kind of tone and texture you had before menopause.

After menstruation has finally ceased, your body is no longer producing any progesterone, although estrogen may still be manufactured by your adrenal glands and fatty tissues. As you have seen, it is progesterone, not estrogen, which awakens the oil-secreting glands within the skin. Without this hormone stimulus, less oil is produced and the skin tends to dry out more quickly. (Dryness results from moisture loss; without an overlying layer of oil to seal them in, the skin's natural fluids evaporate readily.) Older skin is more susceptible to chapping, cracking, infection and fine surface lines because it has lost the moisture-preserving oils that give it its pliability and surface resilience. A woman who takes replacement hormones may be benefiting primarily from progesterone, because this hormone is indirectly associated with oils which have a locally smoothing effect.

(Note: The sun is the *primary* cause of aging skin: It dries out the tissues and inflicts structural damage within the dermis by destroying elastin as well as collagen, the skin's supporting protein, thereby hastening the appearance of permanent wrinkles and sagging.)

As reported in the chapter on menopause, estrogen helps restore drying, thinning vaginal tissues to their moist, originally multi-layered state. Does this mean that the hormone could have the same beneficial effects on the mucous membranes everywhere else? Probably not; after all, the vagina is so sensitive and responsive to estrogen that even when it is topically applied, the hormone has a rejuvenating effect within a relatively short period of time. The same cannot be said for the once-popular estrogen-containing creams slathered on any other part of the body. (They were no more effective locally than an ordinary moisturizer.) Because they have a documented systemic impact, estrogen cosmetic creams have been virtually banned from the market.

While no doctor will or should say that taking replacement hormones will give you younger-looking skin (and this hope alone is *no* reason to embark on such expensive, long-term therapy!) he may point out that your skin can *perhaps* tolerate more dryness if you are on hrt than that of a post-menopausal woman on no therapy. Why? Because hrt mimicks your earlier menstrual cycle and you are still subject to the same hormonal influences that were maintaining your skin before, as a younger woman. If you were prone to oiliness, (a natural camouflage for wrinkles!) you may find you still have to deal with a monthly blemish or two during your progesterone days—although breakouts, if any, are bound to be minimal since you're probably taking far less on a replacement regimen than your own body was producing before. If you always had moist, smooth, problem-free skin then your basic "skinprint" may remain unchanged—a welcome dividend.

REFERENCES AND RECOMMENDED READING

The American Medical Association Book of Womancare by Linda Hughey Holt, M.D. and Melva Webber, Random House, New York, 1982

Clinical Gynecologic Endocrinology and Infertility, Third Edition, by Leon Speroff, Robert H. Glass and Nathan G. Kase, Williams & Wilkins, Baltimore, London, 1982

Dysmenorrhea M. Yusoff Dawood, Editor, Williams & Wilkins, Baltimore, London, 1981

Eve's Journey: The Physical Experience Of Being Female by Susan S. Lichtendorf, G.P. Putnam's Sons, New York, 1982

Freedom From Menstrual Cramps by Dr. Kathryn Schrotenboer and Genell J. Subak-Sharpe, Pocket Books, New York, 1981

Gynecologic Endocrinology, Edited by James Givens, Yearbook Medical Publishers, Chicago, 1977

How To Relieve Cramps and Other Menstrual Problems by Marcia Storch, M.D. and Carrie Carmichael, Workman Publishing, New York 1981

Listen To Your Body by Niels Lauersen, M.D. and Eileen Stukane, Fireside Books (Simon & Schuster), New York, 1982

171

The Ms. Guide To A Woman's Health by Cynthia W. Cooke, M.D. and Susan Dworkin, Doubleday, 1979

Night Thoughts: Reflections Of A Sex Therapist by Avodah K. Offit, M.D., Congdon & Lattes, New York, 1981

No More Hot Flashes & Other Good News by Penny Wise Budoff, M.D., G.P. Putnam's Sons, New York, 1983

Premenstrual Tension by Judy Lever with Dr. Michael G. Brush, McGraw-Hill Book Co., New York, 1981

Sex and The Brain by Jo Durden-Smith and Diane Desimone, Arbor House, New York, 1983

Strictly Female by Carol Ann Rinzler Plume, New York, 1981

Women: A Book For Men Produced by James Wagenwoord and Peyton Bailey, Avon Books, New York, 1979

Index

174

178

About the Authors

Dr. Patricia Allen is an obstetrician/gynecologist in private practice in New York City and clinical instructor in ob/gyn at the College of Physicians and Surgeons, Columbia University. This past year, she has given birth not only to a book but also to a second baby. Dr. Allen is Medical Director of *The Healthy Woman*, a non-profit organization, and has appeared on television as an expert on women's health issues. She lives in Manhattan.

Denise Fortino is health/articles editor at *Harper's Bazaar*, a freelance writer and co-author of *Your Skin: A Dermatologist's Guide To A Lifetime Of Beauty & Health* with Dr. Fredric Haberman, M.D. She is a member of The National Association Of Science Writers and the American Medical Writers Association. Ms. Fortino also lives in New York City.